Taxanes in Lung Cancer Therapy

Taxanes in Lung Cancer Therapy

edited by

David H. Johnson
Vanderbilt University Medical Center
Nashville, Tennessee

Jean Klastersky
Jules Bordet Institute
Brussels, Belgium

MARCEL DEKKER, INC.   NEW YORK · BASEL · HONG KONG

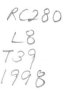

Taxanes in lung cancer therapy/edited by David H. Johnson, Jean Klastersky.
   p. cm.
  Includes index.
  ISBN 0-8247-9892-9 (alk. paper)
  1. Lungs—Cancer—Chemotherapy. 2. Paclitaxel. 3. Docetaxel. I. Johnson, David
H. II. Klastersky, J. (Jean)
  [DNLM: 1. Lung Neoplasms—drug therapy. 2. Paclitaxel—therapeutic use. 3.
Paclitaxel—pharmacology. 4. Carcinoma, Small Cell—drug therapy. 5. Carci-
noma, Non-Small-Cell Lung—drug therapy. WF 658 T235 1998]
RC280.L8T39 1998
616.99'424061—dc21
DNLM/DLC
for Library of Congress   98-11379
                                                     CIP

The publisher offers discounts on this book when ordered in bulk quantities. For more information, write to Special Sales/Professional Marketing at the address below.

This book is printed on acid-free paper.

MARCEL DEKKER, INC.
270 Madison Avenue, New York, New York 10016
http://www.dekker.com

Current printing (last digit):
10 9 8 7 6 5 4 3 2 1

PRINTED IN THE UNITED STATES OF AMERICA

Preface

Lung cancer is the principal cause of cancer-related death in North America and Europe. In the United States alone, more than 165,000 individuals will die of lung cancer in 1997. Sadly, advances in the management of lung cancer have come about slowly and, thus far, have had only minimal impact on the curability of this neoplasm. No more than 15% of all newly diagnosed lung cancer patients survive beyond 5 years, largely because only a small percentage of its victims present with disease that is surgically resectable. For those with unresectable lesions confined to the thorax, the usual treatment consists of radiotherapy alone or in combination with chemotherapy. For those with metastatic disease, treatment is largely palliative and may or may not involve chemotherapy. Some individuals with metastatic disease may derive a survival benefit following chemotherapy, although the survival improvement is modest, averaging just 8 weeks even with the most "effective" drugs currently available.

The dismal results achieved with existing therapies have engendered understandable pessimism among physicians charged with the care of patients with lung cancer. Many physicians question the wisdom of treating patients with metastatic disease and advise against "aggressive" treatments. Fortunately, over the past 5 years, a number of new agents have been identified with good activity against lung cancer. For example, vinorelbine, a compound that interferes with microtubule assembly, has consistently lengthened the life of patients with metastatic non-small-cell lung cancer in randomized trials. More recently, a new class of drugs—the taxanes—have shown considerable promise in the management of lung cancer. The first taxane to enter into clinical trials was paclitaxel, a novel diterpene plant product isolated from the Pacific western yew tree, *Taxus bevifolia*. Paclitaxel produces its cytotoxic effect by promoting the assembly of microtubules and stabilizing their formation by preventing depolymerization. Its congener, docetaxel, works in a similar manner. Both agents are undergoing study throughout the world with encouraging results. Given the promising preliminary results of studies involving this new class of drugs, we compiled the existing data into one useful reference to facilitate the dissemination of these data. *Taxanes in Lung Cancer Therapy* reviews the current knowledge base concerning the use of taxanes in the treatment of lung cancer.

David H. Johnson
Jean Klastersky

Contents

Contributors

W. Akerley, M.D.   Rhode Island Hospital, Providence, Rhode Island

Scott J. Antonia, M.D.   H. Lee Moffitt Cancer Center and Research Institute, Tampa, Florida

H. Anderson, M.D.   Cancer Research Campaign, Department of Medical Oncology, Christie Hospital, Manchester, England

Susan G. Arbuck, M.D.   Head, Developmental Chemotherapy Section, Investigational Drug Branch, Cancer Therapy Evaluation Program, Division of Cancer Treatment and Diagnosis, National Cancer Institute, National Institutes of Health, Bethesda, Maryland

Chandra P. Belani, M.D.   Associate Professor of Medicine, Division of Medical Oncology, Department of Medicine, University of Pittsburgh School of Medicine, and Co-Director, Lung Cancer Program, University of Pittsburgh Cancer Institute, Pittsburgh, Pennsylvania

L. Belli, M.D.   Institut Gustave Roussy, Villejuif, France

Philip Bonomi, M.D.   Director, Section of Medical Oncology, Department of Internal Medicine, Rush University Medical Center, Chicago, Illinois

A. Calderoni, M.D.   Institute of Medical Oncology, Inselspital, Bern, Switzerland

Alan Cantor, M.D.   H. Lee Moffitt Cancer Center and Research Institute, Tampa, Florida

Thomas Cerny, M.D. Professor of Medicine and Oncology, Medical Clinic C, Kantonsspital, St. Gallen, Switzerland

Alex Y. Chang, M.D. Upstate New York Cancer Research and Education Foundation, Rochester, New York

Hak Choy, M.D. Associate Professor, Department of Radiation Oncology, Vanderbilt University Medical Center, Nashville, Tennessee

David S. Ettinger, M.D. Professor of Oncology and Medicine, Associate Director for Clinical Affairs, The Johns Hopkins Oncology Center, Baltimore, Maryland

Ellen G. Feigal, M.D. Clinical Investigation Branch, National Cancer Institute, National Institutes of Health, Bethesda, Maryland

Frank V. Fossella, M.D. Associate Professor and Medical Director, Thoracic Oncology Multidisciplinary Care Center, Department of Thoracic/Head and Neck Medical Oncology, University of Texas M.D. Anderson Cancer Center, Houston, Texas

Linda L. Garland, M.D. Assistant Professor of Medicine, Thoracic Oncology Program, H. Lee Moffitt Cancer Center and Research Institute, Tampa, Florida

Mark S. Georgiadis, M.D. Division of Hematology/Oncology, Department of Internal Medicine, National Naval Medical Center, Bethesda, Maryland

Harvey M. Golomb, M.D. Department of Medicine, University of Chicago Medical Center, Chicago, Illinois

Richard J. Gralla, M.D. Ochsner Clinic, New Orleans, Louisiana

Klaus Havemann, M.D. Professor, Zentrum fur Innere Medizin, Marburg-Lahn, Germany

Mary Heise, M.D. H. Lee Moffitt Cancer Center and Research Institute, Tampa, Florida

Jane Hilstro, M.D. H. Lee Moffitt Cancer Center and Research Institute, Tampa, Florida

Philip C. Hoffman, M.D.   Department of Medicine, University of Chicago Medical Center, Chicago, Illinois

Waun Ki Hong, M.D.   University of Texas M.D. Anderson Cancer Center, Houston, Texas

G. Jayson   Cancer Research Campaign, Department of Medical Oncology, Christie Hospital, Manchester, England

Bruce E. Johnson, M. D.   National Cancer Institute–Navy Medical Oncology Branch, Naval Hospital, Bethesda, Maryland

David H. Johnson, M.D.   Cornelius A. Craig Professor of Medical Oncology and Director, Division of Medical Oncology, Department of Medicine, Vanderbilt University Medical Center, Nashville, Tennessee

T. Le Chevalier, M.D.   Institut Gustave Roussy, Villejuif, France

KyungMann Kim, M. D.   Vanderbilt University Medical Center, Nashville, Tennessee

Jean Klastersky, M.D.   Professor and Chairman, Department of Medicine, Jules Bordet Institute, Brussels, Belgium

Jin Soo Lee, M.D.   University of Texas M.D. Anderson Cancer Center, Houston, Texas

Gregory A. Masters, M.D.   Department of Medicine, University of Chicago Medical Center, Chicago, Illinois

Ann M. Mauer, M. D.   Department of Medicine, University of Chicago Medical Center, Chicago, Illinois

M. Ranson   Cancer Research Campaign, Department of Medical Oncology, Christie Hospital, Manchester, England

O. Rixe, M.D.   Institut Gustave Roussy, Villejuif, France

John C. Ruckdeschel, M.D.   Professor of Medicine and Center Director, H. Lee Moffitt Cancer Center and Research Institute, Tampa, Florida

H. Safran, M.D.   Miriam Hospital, Providence, Rhode Island

J.-P. Sculier, M.D.   Jules Bordet Institute, Brussels, Belgium

Gail Shaw, M.D.   H. Lee Moffitt Cancer Center and Research Institute, Tampa, Florida

Nick Thatcher, Ph.D., F.R.C.P.   Professor, Cancer Research Campaign, Department of Medical Oncology, Christie Hospital, Manchester, England

Everett E. Vokes, M.D.   Professor of Medicine and Radiation Oncology, Department of Medicine, University of Chicago Medical Center, Chicago, Illinois

Henry Wagner, Jr., M.D.   H. Lee Moffitt Cancer Center and Research Institute, Tampa, Florida

Charles C. Williams, Jr., M.D.   H. Lee Moffitt Cancer Center and Research Institute, Tampa, Florida

Martin Wolf, M.D.   Zentrum fur Innere Medizin, Marburg-Lahn, Germany

John J. Wright, M.D., Ph.D.   Investigational Drug Branch, National Cancer Institute, National Institutes of Health, Bethesda, Maryland

Taxanes in Lung Cancer Therapy

1

Taxanes

New Insights into Mechanisms of Drug Action

John J. Wright, Ellen G. Feigal, and Susan G. Arbuck
*National Cancer Institute, National Institutes of Health,
Bethesda, Maryland*

INTRODUCTION

The taxanes paclitaxel and docetaxel are antineoplastic drugs which have novel mechanisms of action that differ from other available anticancer agents. Both compounds are currently prepared from non-cytotoxic precursor molecules extracted from yew species (1,2). The chemical structures of paclitaxel and docetaxel differ at two sites, the 10-position on the baccatin ring and at the 3' position on the lateral chain (Fig. 1).

Both taxanes favor microtubule assembly by reducing the depolymerization of tubulin. They also stabilize formed microtubules (3,4). Docetaxel is twice as potent as paclitaxel with regard to its effect on microtubule depolymerization and slightly more active stabilizing microtubules and promoting tubulin assembly (5,6). Other differences in the drugs that have been noted include the differential modulation of the taxanes by specific microtubule-associated proteins (7) and the structure of tubulin polymer products induced by the two taxanes with regard to protofilament number (8). Despite

1

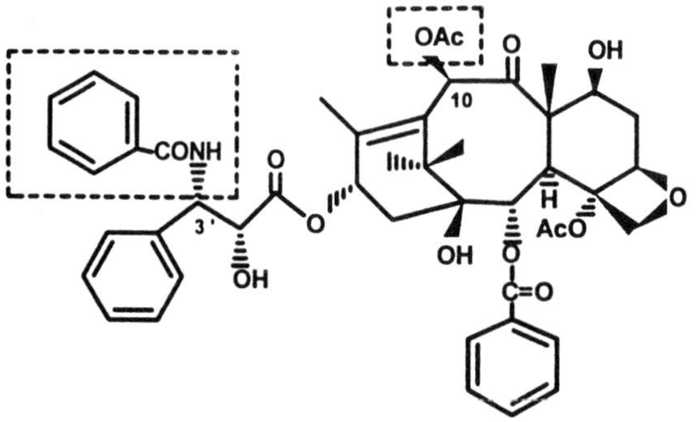

PACLITAXEL (TAXOL®)

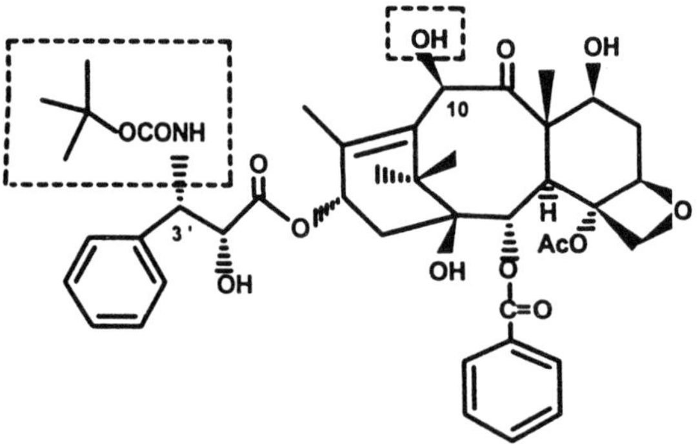

DOCETAXEL (TAXOTERE®)

Figure 1 Chemical structures of paclitaxel and docetaxel.

these differences, both agents are clinically active in a wide variety of tumors.

Microtubules, which are in a state of dynamic equilibrium with their components, the tubulin dimers, are essential components of the mitotic spindle. The taxanes cause interruption of mitotic-specific microtubule processing resulting in mitotic arrest at the G_2-M phase transition. Mitotic arrest has been considered the major mechanism underlying the antineoplasticity of the taxanes (9,10). Microtubules are important in cell division but are also involved in other important cellular functions including the maintenance of cell transmission of signals between cell surface receptors and the nucleus (11). Thus, it is not surprising that altering the equilibrium of the microtubule system can disrupt not only cell division but other normal cellular processes in which microtubules are involved.

Although the broad clinical activity of the taxanes has reaffirmed the importance of microtubules as important targets of anticancer drugs, recent data have suggested that taxane effects are not limited to consequences of their effects on mitosis. Emerging evidence from molecular characterization of taxane-treated cells has provided new insights into the additional effects of these chemotherapeutic agents. While further study and evaluation is essential to elucidate their importance, these preclinical observations may have implications for clinical development of these drugs as antitumor agents. They may be relevant to optimization of dose, to administration schedules, and to combination studies with other chemotherapeutic or biological products. In addition to their effects on mitosis, the broad antitumor activity of the taxanes may be the consequence of effects on the regulation of cell cycle progression, initiation of programmed cell death, and alterations in the expression of gene products critical for tumor angiogenesis, metastasis, or the host immune response. Effects that have been described include:

1. Induction of cell cycle arrest associated with p53-dependent and p53-independent apoptotic cell death.
2. Induction of Bcl-2 phosphorylation and apoptotic cell death by Raf-1-mediated pathway
3. Antimetastatic activity through inhibition of matrix metalloproteinases
4. Inhibition of angiogenesis
5. Alterations of host immunological responses

Many of these processes may be directly or indirectly attributable to microtubule alterations; however, the protean nature of taxane effects suggests that new pathways for mediating the drug's activity may be identified by further study.

TAXANE INDUCTION OF APOPTOSIS

Examination of cell lines in vitro, experimentally transplanted tumors in rodent models (12), and tumor cells from patients undergoing therapy (13) have established that paclitaxel induces morphologic and biochemical changes consistent with apoptosis (14). Human myeloid leukemia cell lines were the first ones shown to undergo apoptosis following exposure to paclitaxel (15) and similar observations were made subsequently with solid tumor cell lines (16–18). The requirement for cellular ATP and inhibition of apoptosis by phosphatases and kinase inhibitors suggested that a process mediated by phosphorylation was requisite for this pathway of paclitaxel cytotoxicity (17–19). Programmed cell death may be induced in HeLa and A549 cell lines with low concentrations of paclitaxel (5 to 10 nM). These concentrations can stabilize microtubule dynamics but do not induce mitotic arrest in G2/M phase (20,21). Recent studies have examined the role of several cellular proteins that are essential for maintaining the complex balance between cellular viability and paclitaxel-induced programmed cell death.

p53

The p53 protein plays a central role in programmed cell death and serves to link the regulation of cell cycle progression with apoptotic pathways. Mutations of this tumor suppressor gene are the most common alteration in human cancers and may serve as a critical initiating event in the transforming process for tumors originating from multiple sites (22). Normal p53 protein binds to specific DNA sequences, such as sites of DNA damage. It blocks progression through the cell cycle and permits repair of DNA damage or allows apoptosis. In contrast, cells with mutant p53 do not arrest and proceed through S-phase with damaged DNA, possibly resulting in uncontrolled cell growth and possibly increasing the risk for subsequent events that lead to cancer (23).

Normal cells express low or undetectable levels of p53, but mutant proteins with a prolonged half-life are detectable. Some studies have suggested that p53 may be a marker for preinvasive neoplasia. Studies using a polyclonal anti-p53 rabbit antiserum detected 90% to 100% nuclear staining in samples from patients with severe lung dysplasia, 100% with in situ or microinvasive cancers, and approximately 40% in samples with mild dysplasia. p53 staining was not detected in squamous metaplasia or in normal lung tissue (24,25).

Inactivation of p53 in some tumors may contribute to radiation and chemotherapy resistance, since the ability to induce apoptotic pathways in these cells in response to DNA-damaging agents is impaired. Such findings have been reported for a variety of standard anticancer agents in a number of experimental systems (26,27). Similarly, results of in vitro studies with the NCI screen, consisting of 60 different human cancer cell lines, demonstrated that most standard anticancer agents are more potent in tumor cells with wild-type p53 (28). In contrast, when paclitaxel was tested against the NCI screen cell lines, the antiproliferative activity of the drug did not correlate with p53 status of the cells.

A similar relationship was noted with a panel of nine human ovarian cancer cell lines that expressed either wild-type p53 (four cell lines), mutant p53 (four cell lines) or had a homozygous deletion (one cell line) of the tumor suppressor gene that prevented expression. The paclitaxel concentration that inhibited growth by 50% was similar in most cell lines and did not correlate with p53 expression status. This was further assessed in two model systems of differential p53 expression using the SKOV 3 human tumor cell line with a homozygous p53 deletion. The introduction of wild-type 053 in an inducible expression vector or a temperature-sensitive mutant of p53 did not alter the cell line's sensitivity to paclitaxel as compared with mock-transfected cells. These results indicate that the cytotoxic activity of paclitaxel in this group of human ovarian cancer cell lines and, at the drug concentration tested (10 nM), proceeded independently of the presence of wild-type or mutant p53 (29).

However, other studies and experimental approaches investigating this relationship between p53 expression and paclitaxel sensitivity have identified alternative outcomes. Normal human fibroblasts that were depleted of functional p53, and primary embryo fibroblasts from p53-null mice were seven- to ninefold more sensitive to paclitaxel cytotoxicity than the parental cell controls with wild-type p53 (30). Disruption of the wild-type p53 gene in an ovarian carcinoma cell line did appear to alter the relative sensitivity to paclitaxel (31). It was proposed that the loss of a p53-induced G1 phase block in these cells allowed cell cycle progression to G2/M, a target stage for paclitaxel-induced cytotoxicity. Thus, there is conflicting evidence on the relative contribution of p53 expression to paclitaxel sensitivity. It is apparent that multiple pathways leading to cell death may be activated by normal and malignant cells following paclitaxel exposure and identifying these differences will be important in establishing the critical factors underlying paclitaxel sensitivity.

Paclitaxel exposure can lead to at least two apoptotic pathways with distinct features. A rapid, p53-independent pathway is induced following arrest of cells in early M at prophase. A slow (3 to 5 days), p53-dependent pathway is induced following a G1 block of cells with wild-type p53 (32). The p53-independent pathway may be very important due to the current paucity of agents with documented efficacy in cells with abnormal or absent p53. Induction of p53 by paclitaxel has been demonstrated in some experimental systems and may activate downstream gene products essential for the programmed cell death program (33).

Bcl-2 Family

Signals that commit cells to continued proliferation or alternative fates are generated by a critical balance between proteins that mediate cell viability and are antiapoptotic, such as Bcl-2 and BCL-x_L, and pro-apoptotic gene products that promote cell death, such as BAX (34). Although Bcl-2 was initially identified in follicular lymphomas with a translocation of chromosomes 14 and 18, the protein is also expressed in SCLC and NSCLC; among the latter, it has been identified in approximately 25% of squamous cell carcinomas and 12% of adenocarcinomas (35,36).

Paclitaxel-induced apoptosis is significantly inhibited in human pre-B leukemia cells transfected with a Bcl-2 expression vector and expressing 10-fold higher levels of the protein than parental cell line. Following exposure to taxol at doses (0.1 nM) that do not induce microtubule bundling or mitotic arrest, the parental cell line underwent apoptosis while the Bcl-2 overexpressing cells were unaffected. The antiapoptotic activity of the increased Bcl-2 expression was relative and could be blunted by higher doses of paclitaxel (37). The taxanes, like other chemotherapeutic agents that affect the integrity of microtubules, alter the critical equilibrium between hypophosphorylated and phosphorylated states of Bcl-2. In human prostate, breast and lymphoid tumor cell lines exposed to paclitaxel or docetaxel, a phosphorylated form of Bcl-2 is expressed (38–40). Phosphorylation inactivates the regulatory function of Bcl-2, possibly by inhibiting heterodimer formation with proapoptotic partners such as BAX, and initiates an apoptotic program in cycling cancer cells. This activity is cell cycle-dependent, requiring transition through the G_2-M phase of the cell cycle.

Docetaxel appears to be effective at inducing Bcl-2 phosphorylation and apoptotic cell death at concentrations almost 100-fold lower than paclitaxel in a panel of human leukemia, lymphoma, and prostate and breast cancer cell lines tested (38).

Bcl-2 phosphorylation following paclitaxel exposure is on a serine residue. Several reports have suggested a role for Raf-1 in the paclitaxel-induced phosphorylation of Bcl-2. Raf-1 is a serine-threonine kinase that acts as a critical intermediate in several pathways connecting membrane-associated tyrosine kinases and Ras with downstream signal transduction pathways (41). Interactions of Raf-1 and Bcl-2 have been shown to be important in some systems for regulation of apoptosis (42). Paclitaxel induces both Raf-1 and Bcl-2 phosphorylation with similar kinetics and drug dose requirements. When Raf-1 is depleted from cells by pretreatment with ansamycin GA, Bcl-2 phosphorylation is inhibited upon subsequent exposure to paclitaxel (43). These experiments support a role for the Raf-1 pathway in phosphorylation of Bcl-2. The paclitaxel-induced phosphorylation of Raf-1 and Bcl-2 appears to be dependent on interaction of the taxane with tubulin and new RNA and protein synthesis (44).

ANTIANGIOGENIC EFFECTS OF TAXANES

Tumor-induced angiogenesis is critical for the growth and progression of solid tumors and has important implications for the metastatic potential of malignant neoplasms. Angiogenesis is a multifaceted process requiring alterations in tumor proliferation and apoptotic activity, expression of endogenous growth factor(s), and migration and invasion by endothelial cells and metastasizing tumor cells. The complexity of this process provides multiple potential target points for intervention with therapeutic agents that may include a number of novel compounds as well as conventional cytotoxic drugs (45).

Several studies have reported that tumor angiogenesis, as represented by microvessel count, may provide prognostic information in non-small-cell lung cancer (NSCLC). In 34 resected NSCLCs, the mean microvessel count, determined by monoclonal antibody staining, was significantly higher in dysplastic epithelium and in situ carcinoma than in normal, hyperplastic, and squamous metaplastic epithelium (46). In 107 early-stage NSCLCs, vascular grade was assessed using the JC70 monoclonal antibody to CD31 (47). Vascular grade and N-stage were not found to be independent prognostic factors by multivariate analysis. However, excluding N-stage, high vascular grade was the only independent prognostic factor for poor survival. In 275 consecutive patients with Stage I NSCLC, patients with higher microvessel numbers had worse survival (48). Multivariate analysis evaluating angiogenesis (microvessel number), protooncogene erbB-2, p53, and proliferation marker Ki-67 identified angiogenesis as the most significant prognostic factor in Stage I NSCLC. In 253 NSCLC patients, tumor microvessel count had the greatest influence on nodal and distant metastasis and patients with high microvessel counts were more likely to die (49). Similar results have been reported in smaller studies in patients with more advanced disease (50) and in other tumor types.

Microtubule inhibitors such as the taxanes, which affect the cytoskeleton, have been identified as inhibitors of angiogenesis using several in vivo and in vitro models. Paclitaxel significantly inhibited the angiogenic response produced by tumor cell supernatant in Matrigel pellets that were subcutaneously implanted in C57BL/6 mice (51). Paclitaxel was also an effective antiangiogenic agent in a model of corneal neovascularization induced by basic fibroblast growth factor (bFGF) or vascular endothelial growth factor (VEGF) (52). In vitro assays assessing various stages of the angiogenesis process also confirmed the antiangiogenic activity of paclitaxel. These studies, which included measurements of endothelial cell proliferation, motility, invasiveness, and cord formation on Matrigel, showed dose-dependent effects of paclitaxel that were not replicated by some other cytotoxic chemotherapeutic agents (e.g., cisplatin, vincristine) (52). The antiangiogenic activity of paclitaxel was distinct from its cytotoxic function. The antiangiogenic activity of paclitaxel may complement the cytotoxic effects of this agent. Efficacy of paclitaxel in the treatment of tumors with a high angiogenic index, such as Kaposi's sarcoma (53,54), may be related to this feature of the drug's activity profile.

ANTIMETASTATIC EFFECTS OF PACLITAXEL

Paclitaxel has been shown to have antimetastatic activity in several preclinical models of tumor metastasis. Several biological processes that are considered to be in vitro correlates of the metastatic phenotype are altered by paclitaxel. In the PC-3 ML prostate cancer cell line, paclitaxel inhibits the production of several proteolytic enzymes that are presumed to be critical for the breakdown of basement membranes, including the type IV collagenases and matrix metalloproteinase II proteins (55). Paclitaxel impairs the translocation of cathepsin B vesicles to the cell periphery and inhibits secretion of this protease, activities that are both dependent on functional microtubular systems (56). Expression of the metastasis-associated gene mts 1 by F1 and BL6 murine melanoma cells is downregulated following paclitaxel exposure (57,58). The drug also has been shown to reduce tumor cell invasion of Matrigel in the Boyden chamber chemotaxis assay and inhibit attachment of PC-3 ML cells (59).

In vivo studies with a SCID mouse model of metastasis established that exposure of PC-3 ML prostate cancer cells to paclitaxel prior to injection or pretreatment of animals with drug before PC-3 ML inoculation, accelerated the clearance of tumor cells from the blood (as measured by assay of circulating ^{125}I-IUDR-labeled tumor cells) and significantly reduced the incidence of bone metastases (60). Prophylactic administration of noncytotoxic paclitaxel doses also significantly inhibited the development of metastases in these animals. The antimetastatic properties of paclitaxel also were tested in the MV522 human NSCLC xenograft model that produces extensive metastases to lung, spleen, and lymph nodes after SC injection in athymic nude mice. Paclitaxel, at toxic doses, was active against the primary tumor but did not reduce metastatic deposits and had an inconsistent impact on median life span (61). The initial results in these model systems of metastasis have been mixed but are nevertheless intriguing and suggest that additional investigations into the antimetastatic potential of the taxanes is warranted. The relative impact of taxane antiangiogenic activity on reducing metastatic tumor progression could also be addressed in these studies.

IMMUNE EFFECTS OF TAXANES

Paclitaxel mimics the actions of endotoxic lipopolysaccharide (LPS) on murine macrophages and activates the antitumor activity of these cells (62,63). Structure/function studies of synthetic analogs of paclitaxel have shown that the benzoyl group at the C-3′ position of the compound is important for this activation process. Structural features of paclitaxel that are essential for binding of the drug to tubulin do not appear to be critical for macrophage activation. This result raises the possibility that the antitumor effect of murine macrophages activated by paclitaxel may not require tubulin polymerization (64).

The LPS-mimetic effects of paclitaxel appear to be under the same genetic control as responses to LPS itself. Both sets of responses are induced only in macrophages from LPS-responsive C3H/OuJ mice and not from the LPS-hyporesponsive C3H/HeJ mouse strain (65). Both LPS and paclitaxel induce protein kinase and cytokine gene cascades in mouse macrophages that lead to expression of new gene products, including nitric oxide synthase (66), arachidonic acid metabolites (20:4) (67), and a subset of early response genes including cytokines (e.g., tumor necrosis factor, granulocyte-macrophage colony-stimulating factor), and transcription factors such as NF-κB (68–71). Preliminary analysis suggests that several different transcriptional and posttranscriptional pathways may be involved in activation of these inducible gene products. Nitric oxide synthase protein expression appears to play a central role in the paclitaxel/LPS activation of murine macrophages (72). The microtubule-disrupting agents colchicine, podophyllotoxin, vinblastine, and nocodazole, which do not have LPS-mimetic effects, inhibit nitric oxide synthase expression (73). Docetaxel, in contrast to paclitaxel, is unable to activate an LPS signal in murine macrophages despite the induction of mitotic arrest and microtubule bundling (74).

The activation of murine macrophage antitumor activity by paclitaxel has been implicated in enhancement of survival in an experimental murine model with the M109 lung adenocarcinoma cell line (75). The identification of a comparable effect in human tumor patients has not been thoroughly evaluated. A preliminary assessment of paclitaxel's effect on human peripheral blood leukocytes did not demonstrate an increase in natural killer cell activity (76). Paclitaxel activates murine macrophages and determining whether similar responses can be achieved in humans will require further study. Since both paclitaxel and docetaxel have substantial clinical activity, the importance of these laboratory observations is not yet clear.

CONCLUSIONS

The taxanes represent an important addition to the chemotherapeutic armamentarium and the full clinical potential of these drugs as conventional cytotoxic agents is still being explored. Paclitaxel originated from the NCI natural products screen but for a variety of reasons was not highly prioritized for development until its novel mechanism of action, polymerizing and stabilizing microtubules, was established. Further studies in the ensuing years have disclosed additional molecular targets that appear to be altered by this class of chemotherapeutic agents. The cytotoxic activity of the taxanes may be mediated by several pathways in addition to the traditional antimitotic pathway originally described. Paclitaxel can induce programmed cell death in a p53-independent manner. Paclitaxel also appears to have antiangiogenic and antimetastatic activity. Antiangiogenic and/or antimetastatic effects may require chronic exposure and presumably would provide maximal benefit in earlier disease stages. It is not yet clear whether taxanes can be administered on a chronic basis at doses that would achieve the desired effects without unacceptable toxicity. Based upon murine studies, paclitaxel may activate the genetic program associated with LPS exposure that unleashes the antitumor potential of immune cells. The relationship of these effects to taxane interactions with microtubules are not fully understood.

The ongoing evaluations of taxane interactions are expected to provide additional intriguing results and may identify evidence of taxane effects on other important biological targets. These findings could eventually lead to additional opportunities to enhance the clinical effectiveness of these drugs. The development of taxane analogs that maximize effects on important molecular targets, particularly those associated with resistance to currently available chemotherapeutic agents, perhaps with less toxicity than the parent compound, might be possible.

REFERENCES

1. Rowinsky EK, Donehower RC. The clinical pharmacology and use of antimicrotubule agents in cancer chemotherapeutics. Pharmacol Ther 1991; 52:35–84.
2. Verweij J, Clavel M, Chevalier B. Paclitaxel (Taxol™) and docetaxel (Taxotere™): not simply two of a kind. Ann Oncol 1994; 5:495–505.
3. Ringel I, Horowitz SB. Studies with RP 56976 (Taxotere): a semi-synthetic analog of taxol. J Natl Cancer Inst 1991; 34:992–998.
4. Pazdur R, Kudelka AP, Kavanagh JJ, et al. The taxoids: paclitaxel (Taxol) and docetaxel (Taxotere). Cancer Treatment Rev 1993; 19:351–386.
5. Gueritte-Voegelein F, Guenard D, Lavelle F, et al. Relationships between the structure of taxol analogues and their anti-mitotic activity. J Med Chem 1991; 34:992–998.

6. Bissery MC, Nohynek G, Sanderink GJ, Lavelle F. Docetaxel (Taxotere®): a review of preclinical and clinical experience. Part I. Preclinical experience. Anticancer Drugs 1995; 6:339–355.

7. Fromes Y, Gounon P, Veitia R, et al. Influence of microtubule-associated proteins on the differential effects of paclitaxel and docetaxel. J Prot Chem 1996; 15:377–388.

8. Andreu JM, Diaz JF, Gil R, et al. Solution structure of Taxotere-induced microtubules to 3-nm resolution. The change in protofilament number is linked to the binding of the taxol side chain. J Biol Chem 1994; 269:31785–31792.

9. Schiff P, Horwitz SB. Taxol stabilizes microtubules in mouse fibroblast cells. Proc Natl Acad Sci USA 1980; 77:1561–1565.

10. Manfredi J, Horwitz SB. Taxol: an antimitotic agent with a new mechanism of action. Pharmacol Ther 1984; 25:83–125.

11. Dustin P. Microtubules. 2nd ed. Berlin: Springer-Verlag, 1984.

12. Milas L, Hunter NR, Kurdoglu B, et al. Kinetics of mitotic arrest and apoptosis in murine mammary and ovarian tumors treated with taxol. Cancer Chemother Pharmacol 1995; 35:297–303.

13. Seiter K, Feldman EJ, Traganos F, et al. Evaluation of in vivo induction of apoptosis in patients with acute leukemia treated on a Phase I study of Paclitaxel. Leukemia 1995; 9:1961–1983.

14. Ireland CM, Pittman SM. Tubulin alterations in taxol-induced apoptosis parallel those observed with other drugs. Biochem Pharmacol 1995; 10:1491–1499.

15. Bhalla K, Ibrado AM, Tourkina E, et al. Taxol induces internucleosomal DNA fragmentation associated with programmed cell death in human myeloid leukemia cells. Leukemia 1993; 7:563–568.

16. Danesi R, Figg WD, Reed E, Myers CE. Paclitaxel (Taxol) inhibits protein isoprenylation and induces apoptosis in PC-3 human prostate cancer cells. Mol Pharm 1995; 47:1106–1111.

17. Liu Y, Bhalla K, Hill C, Priest DG. Evidence for involvement of tyrosine phosphorylation in taxol-induced apoptosis in a human ovarian tumor cell line. Biochemical Pharm 1994; 48:1265–1272.

18. Donaldson KL, Goolsby G, Kiener PA, Wahl AF. Activation of p34[cdc2] coincident with Taxol-induced apoptosis. Cell Growth Diff 1994; 5: 1041–1050.

19. Ponnathpur V, Ibrado AM, Reed JC, et al. Effects of modulators of protein kinases on Taxol-induced apoptosis of human leukemic cells possessing disparate levels of p26 BCL-2 protein. Clin Cancer Res 1995; 1:1399–1406.

20. Jordan MA, Wendell K, Gardiner S, et al. Mitotic block induced in HeLa cell by low concentrations of paclitaxel (Taxol) results in abnormal mitotic exit and apoptotic cell death. Cancer Res 1996; 56:816–825.
21. Torres KE, Castillo G, Horwitz SB. Induction of apoptosis by low concentrations of taxol is not dependent on G2/M block. Proc Am Assoc Cancer Res 1997; 38:530. Abstract 3553.
22. Harris CC. Structure and function of the p53 tumor suppressor gene: clues for rational cancer therapeutic strategies. J Natl Cancer Inst 1996; 88:1442–1455.
23. Denissenko MF, Pao A, Tang M, Pfeiffer GP. Preferential formation of benzo(a)-pyrene adducts at lung cancer mutational hotspots in p53. Science 1996; 274:430–432.
24. Carbone DP, Minna JA. The molecular genetics of lung cancer. Adv Intern Med 1992; 37:153–171.
25. Greenblatt MS, Harris CC. Molecular genetics of lung cancer. Cancer Surv 1995; 25:293–313.
26. Lee JM, Bernstein A. p53 mutations increase resistance to ionizing radiation. Proc Natl Acad Sci USA 1993; 90:5742–5746.
27. Lowe SW, Ruley HE, Jacks T, Housman DE, p53-dependent apoptosis modulates the cytotoxicity of anticancer agents. Cell 1993; 74:957–967.
28. Weinstein JN, Myers TG, O'Connor PM, et al. An information-intensive approach to the molecular pharmacology of cancer. Science 1997; 275:343–349.
29. Debernardis D, Sire EG, De Feudis P, et al. p53 status does not affect sensitivity of human ovarian cancer cell lines to paclitaxel. Cancer Res 1997; 57:870–874.
30. Wahl AF, Donaldson KL, Fairchild C, et al. Loss of normal p53 function confers sensitization to Taxol by increasing G2/M arrest and apoptosis. Nature Med 1996; 2:72–79.
31. Wu GS, El-Deiry WS. P53 and chemosensitivity. Nat Med 1996; 2: 225–226.
32. Woods CM, Zhu J, McQueney PA, et al. Taxol-induced mitotic block triggers rapid onset of a p53-independent apoptotic pathway. Mol Med 1995; 1:506–526.
33. Tishler RB, Lamppu DM, Park S, Price BD. Microtubule-active drugs taxol, vinblastine, and nocodazole increase the levels of transcriptionally active p53. Cancer Res 1995; 55:6021–6025.
34. Rudin CM, Thompson CB. Apoptosis and disease: regulation and clinical relevance of programmed cell death. Annu Rev Med 1997; 48: 267–281.

35. Fontanini G, Vignati S, Bigini D, et al. Bcl-2 protein: a prognostic factor inversely correlated to p53 in non-small-cell lung cancer. Br J Cancer 1995; 71:1003–1007.
36. Walker C, Robertson L, Myskow M, Dixon G. Expression of the BCL-2 protein in normal and dysplastic bronchial epithelium and in lung carcinomas. Br J Cancer 1995; 72:164–169.
37. Tang C, Willingham MC, Reed JC, et al. High levels of p26 BCL-2 oncoprotein retard taxol-induced apoptosis in human pre-B leukemia cells. Leukemia 1994; 8:1960–1969.
38. Haldar S, Basu A, Croce CM. Bcl2 is the guardian of microtubule integrity. Cancer Res 1997; 57:229–233.
39. Haldar S, Jena N, Croce CM. Inactivation of Bcl-2 by phosphorylation. Proc Natl Acad Sci USA 1995; 92:4507–4511.
40. Haldar S, Chintapalli J, Croce CM. Taxol induces bcl-2 phosphorylation and death of prostate cancer cells. Cancer Res 1996; 56:1253–1255.
41. Morrison DK, Cutler RE. The complexity of Raf-1 regulation. Curr Opinion Cell Biol 1997; 9:174–179.
42. Wang H-G, Rapp UR, Reed JC. Bcl-2 targets the protein kinase Raf-1 to mitochondria. Cell 1996; 87:629–638.
43. Blagosklonny MV, Schulte T, Nguyen P, et al. Taxol-induced apoptosis and phosphorylation of Bcl-2 protein involves c-raf-1 and represents a novel c-Raf-1 signal transduction pathway. Cancer Res 1996; 56: 1851–1854.
44. Blagosklonny MV, Giannakakou P, El-Deiry WS, et al. Raf-1/bcl-2 phosphorylation: a step from microtubule damage to cell death. Cancer Res 1997; 57:130–135.
45. Pluda J. Tumor-associated angiogenesis: mechanisms, clinical implications, and therapeutic strategies. Sem Incol 1997; 24:1–18.
46. Fontanini GD, Bigini D, Vignati S, et al. Microvessel count predicts metastatic disease and survival in non-small cell lung cancer. J Pathol 1995; 177:1–18.
47. Giatromanolaki A, Koukourakis M, O'Byrne K, et al. Prognostic value of angiogenesis in operable non-small cell lung cancer. J Pathol 1996; 179:80–88.
48. Harpole DH Jr, Richards WG, Herndon JE, et al. Angiogenesis and molecular biologic substaging in patients with stage I non-small cell lung cancer. Ann Thorac Surg 1996; 61:1470–1476.
49. Fontanini G, Bigini D, Vignati S, et al. Microvessel count predicts metastatic disease and survival in non-small cell lung cancer. J Pathol 1995; 177:57–63.

50. Macchiarini P, Dulmet E, De Montreville V, et al. Prognostic significance of peritumoral blood and lymphatic vessel invasion by tumour cells in T4 non-small cell lung cancer following induction therapy. Surg Oncol 1995; 4:91–99.

51. Belotti D, Vergani V, Drudis T, et al. The microtubule-affecting drug paclitaxel has antiangiogenic activity. Clin Cancer Res 1996; 2:1843–1849.

52. Klauber N, Parangi S, Flynn E, et al. Inhibition of angiogenesis and breast cancer in mice by the microtubule inhibitors 2-methoxyestradiol and taxol. Cancer Res 1997; 57:81–86.

53. Saville MW, Lietzau J, Pluda JM, et al. Treatment of HIV-associated Kaposi's sarcoma with paclitaxel. Lancet 1995; 346:26–28.

54. Karp JE, Pluda JM, Yarchoan R. AIDS-related Kaposi's sarcoma. A template for the translation of molecular pathogenesis into targeted therapeutic approaches. Hematol Oncol Clin North Am 1996; 10: 1031–1049.

55. Stearns ME, Wang M. Immunoassays of the metalloproteinase (MMP-2) and tissue inhibitor of metalloproteinase (TIMP 1 and 2) levels in noninvasive and metastatic PC-3 clones: effects of taxol. Oncol Res 1994; 6:195–201.

56. Rozhin J, Sameni M, Ziegler G, et al. Pericellular pH affects distribution and secretion of cathepsin B in malignant cells. Cancer Res 1994; 54:6517–6525.

57. Parker C, Lakshmi MS, Piura B, et al. Metastasis-associated mts 1 gene expression correlates with increased p53 detection in the B16 murine melanoma. DNA Cell Biol 1994; 13:343–351.

58. Cajone F, Debiasi S, Parker C, et al. Metastasis-associated mts 1 gene expression is down-regulated by heat shock in variant cell lines of the B16 murine melanoma. Melanoma Res 1994; 4:143–150.

59. Stearns ME, Wang M. Taxol blocks processes essential for prostate tumor cell (PC-3ML) invasion and metastases. Cancer Res 1992; 52: 3776–3781.

60. Stearns ME. Taxol reduces circulating tumor cells to prevent bone metastases in SCID mice. Invas Metastasis 1995; 15:232–241.

61. Kelner MJ, McMorris TC, Estes L, et al. Nonresponsiveness of the metastatic human lung carcinoma MV522 xenograft to conventional anticancer agents. Anticancer Res 1995; 15:867–872.

62. Manthey CL, Brandes MB, Perera P-Y, et al. Taxol increases steady-state levels of LPS-inducible genes and protein-tyrosine phosphorylation in murine macrophages. J Immunol 1992; 149:2459.

63. Vogel SN, Manthey CL, Perera PY, et al. Dissection of LPS-induced signaling pathways in murine macrophages using LPS analogs, LPS mimetics, and agents unrelated to LPS. Prog Clin Biol Res 1995; 392: 421–431.

64. Kirikae T, Ojima I, Kirikae F, et al. Structural requirements of taxoids for nitric oxide and tumor necrosis factor production by murine macrophages. Biochem Biophys Res Commun 1996; 227:227–235.

65. Manthey CL, Perera P-Y, Salkowski CA, Vogel SN. Taxol provides a second signal for murine macrophage tumoricidal activity. J Immunol 1994; 152:825–831.

66. Marczin N, Jilling T, Papapetropoulos A, et al. Cytoskeleton-dependent activation of the inducible nitric oxide synthase in cultured aortic smooth muscle cells. Br J Pharmacol 1996; 118:1085–1094.

67. Veis N, Rosen A, Aderem A. Microtubule-active agents mimic lipopolysaccharides in priming macrophages for enhanced arachidonic acid metabolism. J Inflamm 1996; 46:106–113.

68. Henricson BE, Carboni JM, Burkhardt AL, Vogel SN. LPS and Taxol activate Lyn kinase autophosphorylation in Lps(n), but not in Lps(d) macrophages. Mol Med 1995; 4:428–435.

69. Pluznik DH, Lee NS, Sawada T. Taxol induces the hematopoietic growth factor granulocyte-macrophage colony-stimulating factor in murine B-cells by stabilization of granulocyte-macrophage colony-stimulating factor nuclear RNA. Cancer Res 1994; 54:4150–4154.

70. Albrecht H, Schook LB, Jongeneel CV. Nuclear migration of NF-κB correlates with TNF-alpha mRNA accumulation. J Inflamm 1995; 45: 64–71.

71. Perera PY, Qureshi N, Vogel SN. Paclitaxel (Taxol)-induced NF-κB translocation in murine macrophages. Infect Immun 1996; 64:878–884.

72. Jun CD, Choi BM, Kim HM, Chung HT. Involvement of protein kinase C during taxol-induced activation of murine peritoneal macrophages. J Immunol 1995; 154:6541–6547.

73. Kirikae T, Kirikae F, Oghiso Y, Nakano M. Microtubule-disrupting agents inhibit nitric oxide production in murine peritoneal macrophages stimulated with lipopolysaccharide or paclitaxel (Taxol). Infect Immun 1996; 64:3379–3384.

74. Manthey CL, Qureshi N, Stutz PL, Vogel SN. Lipopolysaccharide antagonists block Taxol-induced signaling in murine macrophages. J Exp Med 1993; 178:695–702.

75. Kalechman Y, Shani A, Dovrat S, et al. The antitumoral effect of the immunomodulator AS101 and paclitaxel (Taxol) in a murine model of lung adenocarcinoma. J Immunol 1996; 156:1101–1109.
76. Puente J, Diaz M, Salas MA, et al. Studies of natural killer cell activity in a drug-free, healthy population. Response to a challenge with taxol, estramustine and lipopolysaccharide. Int J Clin Pharmacol 1995; 33: 457–461.

2

In Vitro Testing of Paclitaxel and Docetaxel Against Human Lung Cancer Cell Lines

Implications for Clinical Trials

Mark S. Georgiadis
National Naval Medical Center, Bethesda, Maryland

Bruce E. Johnson
National Cancer Institute–Navy Medical Oncology Branch, Bethesda, Maryland

INTRODUCTION

Paclitaxel and docetaxel are the first members of the new taxane class of chemotherapeutic agents to enter clinical trials and be approved by the Food and Drug Administration (1,2). Interest in paclitaxel as treatment for advanced non-small-cell lung cancer (NSCLC) began with the report of two studies that evaluated paclitaxel as a single agent in a total of 49 chemotherapy naive patients with Stage III or

---

The opinions or assertions herein are the private views of the authors and are not to be construed as official or as reflecting the views of the Department of the Navy or the Department of Defense.

IV disease (3,4). These studies administered paclitaxel at doses of from 200 mg/m^2 to 250 mg/m^2 via 24-h infusion schedules and identified response rates in excess of 20%. More importantly, both studies also found that treated patients had an unusually high 1-year survival rate of approximately 40%. Subsequent Phase II studies of paclitaxel in advanced NSCLC have evaluated either shorter paclitaxel infusion schedules or paclitaxel-containing combination regimens (5–7). Docetaxel as a single agent has also shown significant activity in both previously untreated and platinum-refractory patients with advanced NSCLC (2). In addition, several studies of docetaxel-containing combination regimens in patients with advanced NSCLC have been reported (8–10).

Unfortunately, the most effective paclitaxel infusion schedule and the most active taxane drug combination remain unknown. Several in vitro studies of paclitaxel and docetaxel in lung cancer cell lines have been completed, and these studies may begin to answer some of these questions. In this report, we will review the results of many of these in vitro studies with emphasis on paclitaxel exposure duration and on drug combinations and sequences. In particular, we will present information from studies at the National Cancer Institute–Navy Medical Oncology Branch (NCI–NMOB) that evaluated the schedule-dependent effect of paclitaxel in lung cancer cell lines.

PACLITAXEL SCHEDULE STUDIES

The mechanism of action of the taxane compounds involves an interaction with polymerized tubulin which both promotes the formation and prevents the disassembly of microtubules (1,2). As a consequence, the cytotoxicity of the taxanes is cell cycle-specific with cells being blocked in the G_2/M phase of the cell cycle (11). This cell cycle-specific effect may result in a schedule-dependent effect on cytotoxicity. In particular, longer durations of taxane drug exposure may allow a greater proportion of cells to enter the G_2/M, or susceptible, phase of the cell cycle, and this could result in an increase in cytotoxicity.

Two in vitro studies have evaluated paclitaxel for evidence of a schedule-dependent effect on cytotoxicity in lung cancer cell lines.

Liebmann and colleagues evaluated the lung cancer cell line A549 utilizing a clonogenic assay with paclitaxel exposure durations of 24 to 72 h (12). Above paclitaxel concentrations of 0.05 μM, cytotoxicity was more dependent on increasing durations of exposure rather than increasing paclitaxel concentrations (Fig. 1). In particular, they noted a 100-fold increase in cytotoxicity as exposure duration increased from 24 h to 72 h. In the same report, the authors showed a similar effect for a breast adenocarcinoma (MCF-7) and a pancreatic adenocarcinoma (PC-Sh).

The second study was performed in our laboratories at the NCI–NMOB (13). The NCI–NMOB has established a large number of human lung cancer cell lines from patients in a variety of clinical situations, and previous study has shown that these cell lines exhibit considerable heterogeneity with respect to chemosensitivity testing (14,15). Thus, we evaluated a total of 28 lung cancer cell lines to expand on the concept of the schedule-dependent effect of paclitaxel

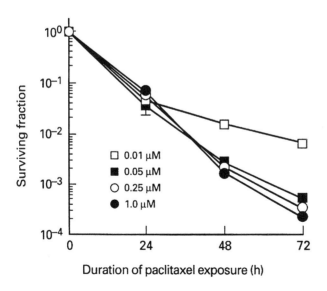

Figure 1 Survival of A549 after exposure to various concentrations of paclitaxel for 24, 48, or 72 hours. From Ref. 12.

Table 1   Median IC_{50} Values (μM) in the MTT Assay for Varying Durations of Paclitaxel Exposure

| | IC_{50} (μM) | | |
| | Exposure duration | | |
Cell lines (n)	3 h	24 h	120 h
NSCLC (14)	>32	16	0.023
SCLC (14)	>32	30	4.5
All lung cancer (28)	>32	24	0.027

cytotoxicity. Fourteen of the cell lines were established from patients with NSCLC, and 14 were from patients with small cell lung cancer (SCLC). Paclitaxel concentrations ranged from 0.0032 μM to 32 μM, and exposure durations were for 3, 24, and 120 h. Cytotoxicity was assessed with the modified tetrazolium-based assay (MTT assay), as previously described (15). The paclitaxel concentration which caused a 50% reduction in cell survival relative to control was defined as the IC_{50}. For the 14 NSCLC cell lines, the median IC_{50} values were >32 μM, 16 μM, and 0.023 μM at exposure durations of 3, 24, and 120 h, respectively (Table 1). For the 14 SCLC cell lines, the median IC_{50} values were > 32 μM, 30 μM, and 4.5 μM, respectively. Six of the 14 SCLC cell lines were very sensitive to paclitaxel, and the median IC_{50} values for these six sensitive SCLC cell lines were > 32 μM, 24 μM, and 0.0032 μM at exposure durations of 3, 24, and 120 h, respectively. Thus, the in vitro, schedule-dependent effect of paclitaxel has been confirmed in separate laboratories utilizing different assay methods. In addition, the effect appears to be consistently present within a broad range of NSCLC cell lines.

DRUG COMBINATION STUDIES

Taxane exposure causes cells to be blocked in the G_2/M phase of the cell cycle, and this cell cycle specificity may in turn result in unique drug-drug interactions (11). In particular, if a taxane compound is combined with an agent that delays or prevents transit through the cell cycle, then the cytotoxicity of the taxane may be reduced. This issue has been addressed with paclitaxel in three in vitro studies utilizing lung cancer cell lines, but, unfortunately, all of these studies were performed in a single cell line, A549. The combinations evaluated were paclitaxel with either doxorubicin, etoposide, cisplatin, or alkylating agents, and all of the studies included an assessment of the sequence of drug exposure.

Akutsu and colleagues studied the combination of paclitaxel and doxorubicin in the human lung adenocarcinoma cell line A549 (16). These investigators assessed cytotoxicity with a modified MTT assay and evaluated the drug interactions by the isobologram method. Cells were incubated with paclitaxel (concentrations up to 0.01 μM) and doxorubicin (concentrations up to 0.02 μM) either simultaneously or sequentially; all drug exposure durations were for 24 h. There was evidence of a less than additive, or antagonistic, effect when the cells were exposed either simultaneously to both agents or to doxorubicin prior to paclitaxel. However, there was evidence of additivity when paclitaxel exposure preceded doxorubicin.

Hahn and colleagues evaluated combinations of paclitaxel with either doxorubicin or etoposide in same cell line, A549 (17). Cells were incubated with paclitaxel, 0.01 μM, for 25 h; during the last hour of incubation, doxorubicin (concentrations up to 5 μg/mL) or etoposide (concentrations up to 50 μg/ml) was added. The reverse sequence was evaluated only with doxorubicin. Cytotoxicity was assessed by the clonogenic assay, and statistical measures of the two-drug combinations were determined by adjusting for cell survival after exposure to a single agent. When paclitaxel preceded either doxorubicin or etoposide, the doxorubicin or etoposide cytotoxicity was less than expected, suggesting a less-than-additive effect of the combination and sequence. However, when doxorubicin exposure preceded paclitaxel incubation, the cytotoxic response was nearly additive up to paclitaxel concentrations of 0.01 μM. These results are in contrast to those of Akutsu et al., but these differences may be related, in part, to differences in assay systems or different models of drug additivity.

Liebmann and colleagues evaluated the combination of paclitaxel and either cisplatin or alkylating agents (melphalan and thiotepa) in the lung cancer cell line A549 (18). They incubated cells for

24 h with paclitaxel 0.1 μM; during the last hour of incubation, cisplatin (concentrations up to 15 μg/mL), melphalan (concentrations up to 16 μg/mL), or thiotepa (concentrations up to 40 μg/mL) were added. Alternatively, cells were initially exposed for 1 h to varying concentrations of cisplatin, melphalan, or thiotepa, washed free of drug, and then incubated for 24 h with paclitaxel 0.1 μM. All drug combinations were additive when paclitaxel preceded cisplatin or either alkylating agent. Conversely, initial treatment with cisplatin or either alkylating agent protected the cells from the effects of paclitaxel, resulting in less than additive cytotoxicity. In the same report, these authors attempted to explain the reason for this sequence-dependent effect. They found that exposure to paclitaxel increased the percentage of cells in the G_2/M phase of the cell cycle from 10% in untreated cell cultures to 86% in paclitaxel-treated cultures. However, pretreatment with cisplatin caused cells to accumulate in S phase, and this potentially protected cells from the cytotoxic effects of paclitaxel.

Preliminary reports of in vitro studies have also addressed the topic of paclitaxel-containing drug combinations and drug sequences. Paclitaxel and carboplatin combinations were evaluated in the lung cancer cell line A549, and the results were similar to the findings with cisplatin (19). Both simultaneous incubation or sequential exposure to paclitaxel followed by carboplatin were more cytotoxic than the sequence of carboplatin followed by paclitaxel. Sequences of paclitaxel and etoposide were also evaluated in A549, and the results were similar to the findings of Hahn and colleagues (20). There was evidence of antagonism when paclitaxel preceded etoposide, but the reverse sequence and simultaneous exposure resulted in synergism.

Similar combination studies with docetaxel in lung cancer cell lines have only been reported in abstract form. Combinations of docetaxel and vinca alkaloids were evaluated in the human lung adenocarcinoma cell line PC-9 (21). The schedule of vinca alkaloid exposure followed by docetaxel resulted in synergism, but the reverse schedule showed antagonism. Other docetaxel combinations were studied in three human lung cancer cell lines (ABC-1, EBC-1, and SBC-3); combinations included docetaxel with etoposide, cisplatin, or vinorelbine (22). Docetaxel and etoposide showed strong antagonism in two of the three cell lines. However, docetaxel with cisplatin showed synergy in two of the three cell lines, and docetaxel with vinorelbine showed synergy in one cell line.

CLINICAL TRIALS

The above in vitro studies served as the basis for our recently completed Phase I clinical trial of paclitaxel by continuous intravenous infusion (CIVI) followed by cisplatin in patients with advanced lung cancer (23). In this trial, 50 patients (42 patients with Stage III/IV NSCLC and 8 patients with extensive-stage SCLC) were treated with up to eight cycles of paclitaxel and cisplatin. Paclitaxel doses ranged from 100 to 180 mg/m^2/96 h and cisplatin doses ranged from 60 to 80 mg/m^2. The maximum tolerated dose (MTD) without granulocyte-colony stimulating factor (G-CSF) support was paclitaxel 120 mg/m^2/96 h and cisplatin 80 mg/m^2, and the MTD with G-CSF support was paclitaxel 160 mg/m^2/96 h and cisplatin 80 mg/m^2. This infusional paclitaxel and cisplatin regimen was active in patients with advanced NSCLC. Thirty-three of the 42 NSCLC patients had measurable disease, and the objective response rate was 55%, with two complete remissions and 16 partial remissions. For all 42 NSCLC patients, the median survival was 10 months, and the actuarial 1-year survival rate was 41%.

Additionally, we studied paclitaxel pharmacokinetics during the first cycle of therapy in this Phase I trial (23). At the MTD without G-CSF, the mean plasma steady-state concentration (Css) of paclitaxel was 0.058 μM (range, 0.040 μM to 0.074 μM), and at the MTD with G-CSF, the mean paclitaxel Css was 0.065 μM (range, 0.053 μM to 0.091 μM). These paclitaxel Css levels are similar to Css levels in other trials administering paclitaxel by prolonged CIVI. Wilson and colleagues administered paclitaxel as a single agent to women with refractory breast cancer; at a paclitaxel dose of 120 mg/m^2/96 h, the Css was 0.053 μM (24). More importantly, our preclinical model of paclitaxel cytotoxicity in lung cancer cell lines showed that the median IC$_{50}$ for the 28 lung cancer cell lines at an exposure duration of 120 h was 0.027 μM (13). Thus, the attainable paclitaxel Css levels in patients treated with prolonged infusions of paclitaxel are greater than the level predicted to be effective in the preclinical model.

Two additional clinical trials have been reported that evaluated the schedule-dependent nature of paclitaxel cytotoxicity. In the first trial, 407 women with platinum-pretreated, relapsed ovarian cancer were randomized to receive one of two doses of paclitaxel at infusion durations of either 3 or 24 h (25). The investigators found no differences in response rates or survival between the women treated with shorter or longer infusion schedule. However, there was considerably more hematological toxicity with the longer infusion schedule. A companion publication evaluated the pharmacokinetic and pharmacodynamic parameters in a subset of these women from the large randomized trial (26). The authors determined that hematologic toxicity did not correlate with the paclitaxel dose, area under the concentration versus time curve, or peak plasma concentration. Rather, toxicity did correlate with duration of exposure to paclitaxel plasma concentrations above a threshold level of 0.05 μM.

The second clinical trial to evaluate the schedule-dependent cytotoxicity of paclitaxel was reported by Seidman and colleagues (27). In this trial, paclitaxel as a single agent via 96-h CIVI was administered to 26 women with metastatic breast cancer refractory to short ($\leq$ 3 h) infusions of taxanes. Seven of 26 patients (27%) responded to the prolonged paclitaxel infusion after failing the shorter infusion. These clinical data, when combined with the results of the in vitro studies previously described, suggest that paclitaxel is a schedule-dependent agent and that both hematologic toxicity and cancer cell cytotoxicity are increased with longer paclitaxel exposure durations. Such a schedule-dependent effect is not unique to paclitaxel. A similar effect has been confirmed for etoposide via both in vitro studies and a subsequent randomized clinical trial (28,29).

SUMMARY

The cytotoxic effect of paclitaxel is schedule-dependent with longer in vitro incubations resulting in greater cytotoxicity. This effect is independent of the assay system, and the effect is consistent in a broad range of NSCLC cell lines. These in vitro data formed the basis for the Phase I clinical trial evaluating a 96-h paclitaxel infusion in combination with cisplatin for patients with advanced lung cancer. The results of this clinical trial are encouraging, but, contrary to the in vitro predictions, the regimen does not appear to be an order of magnitude more active against lung cancer than regimens that include conventional (3- to 24-h) paclitaxel infusions (3–7). It is possible that clinical trials with paclitaxel infusions even longer than 96 h will be required to fully address this schedule issue.

In addition, the combination of either paclitaxel or docetaxel with a platinum compound is at least additive in multiple in vitro models, and the combination is sequence-dependent. Phase I and Phase II clinical trials have begun to evaluate paclitaxel/platinum combinations in patients with advanced lung cancer and have yielded promising results (7,23). Several in vitro models, however, show evidence of antagonism with the combination of either paclitaxel or docetaxel and etoposide, and in vitro studies of the combination of paclitaxel and doxorubicin yield conflicting results. These studies, however, are all limited because they utilize a single human lung cancer cell line, A549. Additional in vitro studies should evaluate taxane drug combinations in a number of cell lines and should utilize rigorous measurements of drug interactions to determine if the conclusions can be broadly applied in clinical trials.

REFERENCES

1. Rowinsky EK, Donehower RC. Drug therapy: paclitaxel (Taxol). N Engl J Med 1995; 332:1004–1014.
2. Cortes JE, Pazdur R. Docetaxel. J Clin Oncol 1995; 13:2643–2655.
3. Murphy WK, Fossella FV, Winn RJ, et al. Phase II study of taxol in patients with untreated advanced non-small-cell lung cancer. J Natl Cancer Inst 1993; 85:384–388.
4. Chang AY, Kim K, Glick J, et al. Phase II study of taxol, merbarone, and piroxantrone in stage IV non-small-cell lung cancer: the Eastern Cooperative Oncology Group results. J Natl Cancer Inst 1993; 85: 388–394.

5. Millward MJ, Bishop JF, Friedlander M, et al. Phase II trial of a 3-hour infusion of paclitaxel in previously untreated patients with advanced non-small-cell lung cancer. J Clin Oncol 1996; 14:142–148.

6. Hainsworth JD, Thompson DS, Greco FA. Paclitaxel by 1-hour infusion: an active drug in metastatic non-small-cell lung cancer. J Clin Oncol 1995; 13:1609–1614.

7. Langer CJ, Leighton JC, Comis RL, et al. Paclitaxel and carboplatin in combination in the treatment of advanced non-small-cell lung cancer: a Phase II toxicity, response, and survival analysis. J Clin Oncol 1995; 13:1860–1870.

8. Cole JT, Gralla RJ, Marques CB, et al. Phase I-II study of cisplatin + docetaxel (Taxotere) in non-small cell lung cancer. Proc Annu Mtg Am Soc Clin Oncol 1995; 14:A1087.

9. Zalcberg JR, Bishop JF, Millward MJ, et al. Preliminary results of the first Phase II trial of docetaxel in combination with cisplatin in patients with metastatic or locally advanced non-small cell lung cancer. Proc Annu Mtg Am Soc Clin Oncol 1995; 14:A1062.

10. Le Chevalier T, Belli L, Monnier A, et al. Phase II study of docetaxel (Taxotere) and cisplatin in advanced non-small cell lung cancer: an interim analysis. Proc Annu Mtg Am Soc Clin Oncol 1995; 14:A1059.

11. Liebmann J, Cook JA, Lipschultz C, et al. The influence of Cremophor EL on the cell cycle effects of paclitaxel (Taxol) in human tumor cell lines. Cancer Chemother Pharmacol 1994; 33:331–339.

12. Liebmann JE, Cook JA, Lipschultz C, et al. Cytotoxic studies of paclitaxel (Taxol) in human tumour cell lines. Br J Cancer 1993; 68:1104–1109.

13. Georgiadis MS, Russell E, Johnson BE. Prolonging the exposure of human lung cancer cell lines to paclitaxel increases the cytotoxicity. Lung Cancer 1994; 11(suppl 1):95. Abstract.

14. Phelps RM, Johnson BE, Ihde DC, et al. The NCI-Navy Medical Oncology Branch cell line data base. J Cell Biochem 1996; 24(suppl):32–91.

15. Carmichael J, Mitchell JB, DeGraff WG, et al. Chemosensitivity testing of human lung cancer cell lines using the MTT assay. Br J Cancer 1988; 57:540–547.

16. Akutsu M, Kano Y, Tsunoda S, et al. Schedule-dependent interaction between paclitaxel and doxorubicin in human cancer cell lines in vitro. Eur J Cancer 1995; 31A:2341–2346.

17. Hahn SM, Liebman JE, Cook J, et al. Taxol in combination with doxorubicin or etoposide: possible antagonism in vitro. Cancer 1993; 72:2705–2711.

18. Liebmann JE, Fisher J, Teague D, et al. Sequence dependence of paclitaxel (Taxol) combined with cisplatin or alkylators in human cancer cells. Oncol Res 1994; 6:25–31.

19. Clark JW, Santos-Moore AS, Choy H. Sequencing of Taxol and carboplatin therapy. Proc Annu Mtg Am Assoc Cancer Res 1995; 36: A1772.

20. Perez EA, Hack F, Fletcher T. Sequence dependent cytotoxicity of Taxol and etoposide in lung and breast human cancer cell lines. Proc Annu Mtg Am Soc Clin Oncol 1995; 14:A1604.

21. Hino M, Kobyashi K, Hayashihara K, et al. In vitro combination effect of docetaxel (RP56976) with vinca alkaloids on cancer cell lines. Proc Annu Mtg Am Assoc Cancer Res 1995; 36:A1780.

22. Aoe K, Ueoka H, Kiura K, et al. Synergistic effect of docetaxel and vinorelbine against in vitro growth of a human small-cell lung cancer cell line. Proc Annu Mtg Am Assoc Cancer Res 1996; 37:A2560.

23. Georgiadis MS, Schuler BS, Brown JE, et al. Paclitaxel by 96-hour continuous infusion in combination with cisplatin: a Phase I trial in patients with advanced lung cancer. J Clin Oncol 1997; 15:735–743.

24. Wilson WH, Berg SL, Bryant G, et al. Paclitaxel in doxorubicin-refractory or mitoxantrone-refractory breast cancer: a Phase I/II trial of 96-hour infusion. J Clin Oncol 1994; 12:1621–1629.

25. Eisenhauer EA, Huinink WW, Swenerton KD, et al. European-Canadian randomized trial of paclitaxel in relapsed ovarian cancer: high-dose versus low-dose and long versus short infusion. J Clin Oncol 1994; 12:2654–2666.

26. Gianni L, Kearns CM, Giani A, et al. Nonlinear pharmacokinetics and metabolism of paclitaxel and its pharmacokinetic/pharmacodynamic relationships in humans. J Clin Oncol 1995; 13:180–190.

27. Seidman AD, Hochhause D, Gollub M, et al. Ninety-six-hour paclitaxel infusion after progression during short taxane exposure: a Phase II pharmacokinetic and pharmacodynamic study in metastatic breast cancer. J Clin Oncol 1996; 14:1877–1884.

28. Wolff SN, Grosh WW, Prater K, et al. In vitro pharmacodynamic evaluation of VP-16-213 and implications for chemotherapy. Cancer Chemother Pharmacol 1987; 19:246–249.

29. Slevin ML, Clark PI, Joel SP, et al. A randomized trial to evaluate the effect of schedule on the activity of etoposide in small-cell lung cancer. J Clin Oncol 1989; 7:1333–1340.

3

Phase II Trials with Paclitaxel in Non-Small-Cell Lung Cancer

North American Experience

Alex Y. Chang
Upstate New York Cancer Research and Education Foundation,
Rochester, New York

INTRODUCTION

Paclitaxel is a novel natural product with unique mechanisms of action and structure. Encouraging antitumor activities have been observed with paclitaxel in preclinical and Phase I studies against non-small-cell lung cancer (1,2). Phase II trials in non-small-cell lung cancer were not initiated until the late 1980s due to scarce supply and the observation of hypersensitivity reactions and cardiac arrhythmia caused by paclitaxel. Once the hurdle of hypersensitivity reaction was overcome by premedication of steroids and antihistamines, Phase II trials were started with the National Cancer Institute (NCI)-recommended dose of 200 to 250 mg/m^2 over 24-h infusion. Since the promising results of Phase II studies using this schedule were reported, other doses and schedules have also been evaluated. This section will describe the North American (including Australian) experience of Phase II trials with paclitaxel in chemotherapy-naive advanced non-small-cell lung cancer patients. Patients with prior chemotherapy will be dealt with in a later section.

DESCRIPTION AND SUMMARY OF PHASE II TRIALS

Table 1 summarizes the results, dose, and schedules of paclitaxel Phase II trials in non-small-cell lung cancer. The treatment interval varies from weekly to every 3 weeks, and dose ranges from 100 mg to 250 mg. The infusion duration of chemotherapy also ranges widely from 1 h to 24 h. Table 1 also shows that the lower dose intensity of paclitaxel may have a lower response rate.

The treatment results of the Eastern Cooperative Oncology Group (3) and the M.D. Anderson Cancer Center (4) are very consistent with each other as to response rate (21% vs. 24%), 1-year survival rate (42% vs. 38%), and toxicity profile. The major dose-limiting toxicity is the high frequency (67% to 96%) of grade IV neutropenia in patients treated with 24-h infusion of paclitaxel in both studies. Both suggest the use of granulocyte colony-stimulating factor (G-CSF) to ameliorate the myelosuppression from this schedule of paclitaxel.

Table 1   Results of Phase II Trials with Paclitaxel in Non-Small-Cell Lung Cancer: North American Experience

	Dose mg/m^2	Schedule	Infusion duration	No. of patients	CR + PR	1 year survival
Chang et al. (3) (ECOG)	250	q3wk	24 h	24	21%	42%
Murphy et al. (4) (M.D. Anderson)	200	q3wk	24 h	25	24%	38%
Millward et al. (5) (Australia)	175	q3wk	3 h	51	10%	40%
Hainsworth et al. (6) (Nashville, TN)	135	q3wk	1 h	17	12%	
	200	q3wk	1 h	42	31%	33%
Akerley et al. (7) (Rhode Island Hospital)	100–200	Weekly × 6 q8wk	3 h	24	38%	NA

In the Millward trial (5), paclitaxel (Anzatax, Faulding) was given over 3-h infusion at 175 mg/m^2 every 3 weeks. It had the largest patient population, 51, and reported only a 10% response rate. This trial included performance status two patients, and showed a different toxicity pattern from those in Chang's (3) and Murphy's (4) studies. Millward et al. reported that 22% of patients had grade 3 or 4 myalgia and arthralgia, and only 16% had grade 4 neutropenia. The poor result can be explained partly by the inclusion of performance status two patients, as well as the lower dose of paclitaxel.

Hainsworth's trial (6) reported a 12% response rate in patients treated with 1-h paclitaxel infusion of 135 mg/m^2 and a 31% response rate of 200 mg/m^2 ($P < .5$). Although this was not a randomized study, it suggests that a dose-response relationship may exist between the dose of paclitaxel and the clinical response on a given schedule. Other results worth noting from the same trial are that six of 16 patients (38%) who failed a cisplatin-based regimen responded to 200 mg/m^2 of paclitaxel and only 12% had grade 3 or 4 leukopenia, suggesting that paclitaxel and cisplatin are not cross-resistant. Both Millward's and Hainsworth's trials also showed that shorter infusion time of paclitaxel had less myelosuppression than longer infusion time.

This brings us to the most intriguing trials reported recently by Akerley et al. (7), who observed a 38% response rate in 24 patients treated with 3-h infusion weekly for 6 weeks with 2 weeks rest at a dose of 100 to 200 mg/m^2 with reasonable toxicity profiles.

Again, Akerley's study suggests that the paclitaxel dose intensity can be increased two- to threefold with reduced toxicity despite the fact that seven patients in their trial had a performance status of 2. Neurotoxicity as well as neutropenia became dose-limiting at a dose of 200 mg/m^2/week, and they have suggested 175 mg/m^2/week for future Phase II trials.

All five trials, although they involved a small number of patients and were Phase II studies without randomized controls, suggest that the clinical activity of paclitaxel in patients with advanced non-small-cell lung cancer depends on the infusion duration, dose intensity, and treatment intervals. The trend is toward higher dose intensities producing higher response rates. It is also important to point out that different treatment schedules produced different side effects. Further clinical trials may shed light on the optimal schedule, dose, and intervals for selected subsets of patients such as the elderly or those with poor performance status.

DISCUSSION

Chang's (3) and Murphy's (4) report established that paclitaxel with 24-h infusion every 3 weeks between 200 and 250 mg/m^2 is among the most active single agents in the treatment of non-small-cell lung cancer. The 1-year actuarial survival rate of 40% in both trials is the first indication that paclitaxel may improve the survival of this group of patients as compared to the historical control of 20% to 25% survival rate in patients treated with cisplatin and etoposide (8,9). Although the combination of paclitaxel and cisplatin is superior to etoposide and cisplatin in the treatment of metastatic non-small-cell lung cancer (10), whether treatment with paclitaxel alone will produce a superior survival rate to treatment with etoposide and cisplatin or equivalent to paclitaxel and cisplatin awaits further randomized clinical trials.

From our own in vitro studies of paclitaxel against A549 adenocarcinoma of lung cancer cells (11) as well as other in vitro studies (1,12,13), the most important determining factor for cytotoxicity is the time of exposure. Paclitaxel can be very effective in producing one log cell kill of A549 cells with a concentration of 10 nM as long as the exposure time is longer than 24 h (11). Most of the clinical pharmacology studies suggest that even in doses below 100 mg/m^2, paclitaxel serum levels will be over 10 nM. However, how long the blood level is sustainable at or above 10 nM is not usually reported. Missing from the list of trials in Table 1 is 96-h infusion at 35 mg/m^2/day or even longer duration of infusion time such as 7 to 21 days. It is not clear whether 96-h infusion or longer duration of infusion will result in a better response in patients with non-small-cell lung cancer (NSCLC). The maximum tolerated dose by 96-h infusion was determined to be 140 mg/m^2 in patients with prior chemotherapy (14), and responses have been seen in patients with disease refractory to short duration of taxane infusion. We have observed two of 12 patients with NSCLC who had not responded to 3-h paclitaxel infusion at 135 mg/m² every 3 weeks responded to 96-h continuous infusion of paclitaxel at the same total dose. Similar observations were made by Siedman (15) and Chang et al. (16). They reported respectively that 7/26 and 3/5 patients with metastatic breast cancer responded to 96-h paclitaxel infusion after their disease had become refractory to short infusion of taxane. This phenomenon suggests that mechanism of resistance developed by tumor cells to short infusion (1 to 3 h) of paclitaxel may be partially reversed by 96-h infusion of paclitaxel. This, in turn, may just simply be due to longer exposure time of paclitaxel or to a different cytotoxic mechanism in operation. The latter notion is supported by the recent report that low concentration of paclitaxel has a different mechanism of action from stabilizing the microtubule mass (17). This is very similar to the situation of 5-fluorouracil (18,19).

These clinical observations are consistent with preclinical studies that prolonged paclitaxel exposure time has a greater cytotoxicity than increasing the concentration (1–2,11–13). In agreement with the above conclusion, Siedman et al. (15) reported that the steady-state serum concentration of paclitaxel does not correlate with response but does correlate with neutropenia.

In addition to infusion time of paclitaxel, the other factor that may influence response is dosage. It seems that at the same infusion time and treatment interval (especially shorter infusion time, such as 1 h or 3 h), the higher the dose of paclitaxel, the higher the response rate. This may indicate that there may exist a threshold for response to paclitaxel which would be consistent with nonlinear pharmacokinetic data when paclitaxel is given in a short infusion time (1,5).

It is also interesting to note that six of 16 patients (38%) responded to paclitaxel by 1-h infusion at 200 mg/m²/week after the disease had failed to respond to cisplatin-containing regimens. This suggests that paclitaxel and cisplatin are not completely cross-resistant. Cisplatin and paclitaxel are synergistic in preclinical studies (2). Thus, a combination of the two agents may hold greater promise for patients with metastatic non-small-cell lung cancer and should warrant further studies with various schemata of combinations of the two.

Without further studies it is impossible to conclude that paclitaxel should be used in patients with performance status 2 or worse or in elderly patients (> 70 years old). Whether such patients should receive chemotherapy for their metastatic non-small-cell lung cancer is also open to debate. One will need to define a nontoxic and effective regimen for this group of patients. Weekly vinorelbine (20) and weekly paclitaxel are potential candidates and warrant further study.

CONCLUSION

Paclitaxel as a single agent is an effective treatment in chemotherapy-naive patients with advanced non-small-cell lung cancer. Defining the optimal schedule, dose, and infusion time will require further randomized controlled studies. Higher dose and longer or more frequent exposure of patients to effective cytotoxic concentrations may yield a higher response rate and less toxicity or a different toxicity pattern. Whether paclitaxel combinations will be better than paclitaxel alone in this disease also awaits further trials.

REFERENCES

1. Rowinsky EK, Cazenave LA, Donehower RC. Taxol: a novel investigational antimicrotubule agent. JNCI 1990; 82:1247–1259.
2. Ross WC. Taxol-based combination chemotherapy and other in vivo preclinical antitumor studies. JNCI 1993; 15:47–53.
3. Chang AY-C, Kim K, Glick J, et al. Phase II study of taxol, Merbarone and piroxantrone in Stage IV non-small cell lung cancer: the Eastern Cooperative Oncology Group results. JNCI 1993; 85:384–387.
4. Murphy WK, Fossella FV, Winn RJ, et al. Phase II study of taxol in patients with untreated advanced non-small cell lung cancer. JNCI 1993; 85:384–387.
5. Millward MJ, Bishop JF, Friendlander M, et al. Phase II trial of a 3-hour infusion of paclitaxel in previously untreated patients with advanced non-small cell lung cancer. J Clin Oncol 1996; 14:142–148.

6. Hainsworth JD, Thompson DS, Greco FA. Paclitaxel by 1-hour infusion: an active drug in metastatic non-small cell lung cancer. J Clin Oncol 1995; 13:1609–1614.
7. Akerley W, Choy H, Glantz M, et al. Weekly paclitaxel for metastatic non-small cell lung cancer: a phase I trial. Proc Am Soc Clin Oncol 1996; 15:377. Abstract.
8. Klastersky J, Sculier JP, Lacroix H, et al. A randomized study comparing cisplatin or carboplatin with etoposide in patients with advanced non-small cell lung cancer: European Organization for Research and Treatment of Cancer protocol 07861. J Clin Oncol 1990; 8:1556–1562.
9. Idhe DC, Minna JD. Non-small cell lung cancer. II. Treatment. Curr Prob Cancer 1991; 15:105–154.
10. Bonomi P, Kim K, Chang A, Johnson D. Phase III trial comparing etoposide-cisplatin versus taxol with cisplatin-G-CSF versus taxol-cisplatin in advanced non-small cell lung cancer. An Eastern Cooperative Oncology Group trial. Proc Am Soc Clin Oncol 1996; 15:382. Abstract.
11. Chang AY. Paclitaxel in the treatment of non-small cell lung cancer. In: McGuire W, Rowinsky EK, eds. Paclitaxel in Cancer Treatment. New York: Marcel Dekker, 1995:273–279.
12. Lopes NM, Adams EG, Pitts TW, et al. Cell kill kinetics and cell cycle effects of taxol on human and hamster ovarian cell lines. Cancer Chemother Pharmacol 1993; 32:235–242.
13. Liebmann JE, Cook JA, Lipschultz C, et al. Cytotoxic studies of paclitaxel (Taxol) in human tumor cell lines. Br J Cancer 1993; 68:1104–1109.
14. Wilson WH, Berg S, Bryant G, et al. Paclitaxel in doxorubicin-refractory or mitoxantrone-refractory breast cancer: a phase I/II trial of 96-hour infusion. J Clin Oncol 1994; 12:1621–1629.
15. Seidman AD, Hochhauser D, Gollub M, et al. Ninety-six-hour paclitaxel infusion after progression during short taxane exposure: a phase II pharmacokinetic and pharmacodynamic study in metastatic breast cancer. J Clin Oncol 1996; 14:1877–1884.
16. Chang AY, Boros L, Garrow G, Asbury R. Paclitaxel by 3-hour infusion followed by 96-hour infusion on failure in patients with refractory malignant disease. Semin Oncol 1995; 22(suppl 6):124–127.
17. Jordan MA, Toso RJ, Thrower D, Wilson L. Mechanism of mitotic block and inhibition of cell proliferation by Taxol at low concentration. Proc Natl Acad Sci USA 1993; 90:9552–9556.
18. Lokich J, Anderson N. Infusional cancer chemotherapy: historical evolution and future development at the Cancer Center of Boston. Cancer Invest 1995; 13:202–226.

19. Aschele A, Sobrero A, Faderan MA, et al. Novel mechanisms of resistance to 5-fluorouracil in human cancer sublines following exposure to two different clinical relevant dose schedules. Cancer Res 1992; 52: 1855–1864.
20. Gridelli C, DeMarinis F, Ianiello G, et al. Phase II study of vinorelbine in elderly patients with stage III$_B$-IV non-small cell lung cancer: activity, symptoms' relief and optimal schedule. Proc Am Soc Clin Oncol 1996; 15:392. Abstract.

4

Phase II Results of Taxanes in Lung Cancer

European Experience

Thomas Cerny
Medical Clinic C, Kantonsspital, St. Gallen, Switzerland

A. Calderoni
Institute of Medical Oncology, Inselspital, Bern, Switzerland

INTRODUCTION

After a decade without the introduction of new cytotoxic drugs for lung cancer, several new drugs are now available with consistent activity. Among the classes of new agents, the taxanes (paclitaxel and docetaxel) play a major role. Their target is the cytoplasmic microtubule, and, contrary to the well-known vinca alkaloids, they rather prevent than promote this assembly eventually interrupting the process of cell division. Taxoids are extracts from the pacific (paclitaxel) or the European (docetaxel) yew tree. Docetaxel (Taxotere®) differs from paclitaxel (Taxol®) in two separate positions on the taxane ring structure. These drugs are insoluble in water and require preparation in lipophilic solvent. Activity has been found in small- (SCLC) and non-small-cell (NSCLC) lung cancer. The activity of the new agents alone or combination continues to be a topic of great clinical importance. Their role in neoadjuvant approach of chemotherapy followed by surgical resection has to be defined.

RESULTS

Phase II Results of Paclitaxel (Taxol) in NSCLC

Short infusions of 1–3 h of paclitaxel (Taxol) at a dose of 225 mg/m^2 showed PR in 18% to 24% in 105 patients with NSCLC (10,11). At the dose of 250 mg/m^2 given as a continuous infusion for 24 h the activity was very similar with a PR of 21% to 24% in a total of 49 patients (8,9). Neither schedule yielded complete remission, but length of median survival of 53 weeks (9) was exceptionally good. Toxicity showed no unusual pattern as compared to other Phase II studies, with hematological toxicity and consecutive infections being the major dose-limiting toxicity (Table 1).

These promising results initiated a large series of phase II combination regimens with cisplatin (Platinol®) or carboplatin. In these combinations paclitaxel (Taxol) was given at a dose of 135 to 215 mg/m^2 as a 24-h infusion in combination with carboplatin (9,20,21) and the overall response was between 27% to 62% with a CR rate up to 9%.

Since the 3-h infusion is more attractive for clinical use than the 24-h schedule, many more trials looked at the 3-h paclitaxel (Taxol) infusion with platinum analogs. The dosage used was 110 to 225

Table 1   NSCLC, Single-Agent Paclitaxel (Taxol)

Reference	Pts	Dose mg/m^2	Adeno/ squamous/ others %	Prior Rx	PR (%)	CR (%)	Note
Chang (8)	24	250 (24 h inf)	42/25/34	No	21%	0	1-year surv 41%
Murphy (9)	25	250 (24 h inf)	68/12/20	No	24%	0	53 weeks median surv
Gatzemeier (10)	50	225 (1–3 h inf)	NS	No	24%	0	
Hainsworth (11)	55	225 (1–3 h inf)	NS	No	18%	0	

mg/m^2 and the overall response rate varied from 26% to 52% with CRs of up to 12%. Toxicity was mainly hematological, but neuro-toxicity was the dose-limiting side effect in some patients with the cisplatinum combination. Interestingly, the expected cumulative hematological toxicity of the combination with carboplatin was not found, and there seemed to be a bone marrow-protective effect of this particular combination. This interesting finding is now under further careful evaluation (Table 2a).

A further attempt has been made to shorten paclitaxel (Taxol) application to only 1 h, and results were very comparable to the other schedules (37,39,40,47,48,52). The study of Hainsworth (46) included a third drug, and patients received a radiotherapy of 60 Gy after two cycles with concomitant dose-adapted chemotherapy. An overall response rate of 72% was found with a CR rate of 36%. Median survival exceeded 12 months (Table 2b).

Since inoperable non-small-cell lung cancer Stage III patients usually respond better than more advanced Stage IV patients, the results of paclitaxel (Taxol) in Stage III patients only are of great importance. These patients might be candidates for neoadjuvant strategies in order to get a curative chance. Three studies (34,41,42) in combination with platinum analogs and/or etoposide (34,41) showed a high response rate, of 63% to 68%, and even 86% in the study of Choy (42) where Taxol 60 mg/m^2 was given weekly for 6 weeks followed by radiotherapy 60 Gy in a total of 33 patients. These results are highly promising for future studies including all three classical therapeutic modalities such as chemotherapy, radiotherapy, and surgery (Table 2c).

Phase II Results of Docetaxel (Taxotere) in NSCLC

Taxotere (docetaxel) is a semisynthetic taxoid prepared from a non-cytotoxic precursor extracted from the needles of the European yew tree (*Taxus baccata*). Twelve studies have addressed the question of activity of docetaxel (Taxotere) single-agent therapy of non-small-cell lung cancer of all subtypes with an OR of 17% to 38% and even one CR (12). Median survival was again close to 1 year. The dose of docetaxel (Taxotere) was 60 to 100 mg/m^2 and usually given over 1 h.

Table 2a Combinations with Paclitaxel

Time Ref.	Pts	Prior Rx	Paclitaxel mg/m²	Other agents	Adeno/ squamous/ other %	PR	CR	PR+ CR	Notes
24-h									
Langer (19)	53	No (15% had RT)	135–215	CBDA AUC 7.5	65/22/13	28 (53%)	5 (9%)	33 (62%)	Median surv > 52 weeks! 1 year surv of 54%
Belani (20)	26	No	135,175, 200	CBDA AUC 6 to 7.5	NS	12 (46%)	1 (4%)	13 (50%)	
Johnson (21)	51	No	135,175	CBDA AUC 6	73/12/15	14 (27%)	0	14 (27%)	
3-h									
Kosmidis (24)	42	No	175	CBDA AUC 7	30/?/?	11 (26%)	0	11 (26%)	
Von Pawel (25)	67	No	175	CDDP 75	NS	25 (37%)	3 (5%)	28 (42%)	Median surv 10 month
Steppert (28)	18[a] 26	No	200	CBDA 300– 350	NS	NS	NS	6 (33%) 13 (50%)	
Sorensen (35)	30[b] 19 eval	No	110	CDDP 60	53/?/?	F8 (42%)	1 (5%)	9 (47%)	
Schütte (38)	25	No	200	CBDA AUC 5.0	24/40/36	10 (40%)	3 (12%)	13 (52%)	
Belli (49)	32 29 eval	No	135–225	CDDP 100	62/13/25	11 (38%)	0	11 (38%)	

1-h

					75/?/?				
Langer (37)	32 22 eval	No	175–280	CBDA AUC 7.5	75/?/?	12 (55%)	0	12 (55%)	Median surv > 12 mo
Roa (39)	18	Yes	200 (1–3 h)	CBDA AUC 5.0	NS	0	0		
Roa (40)	14	No	200 (1–3 h)	CBDA AUC 6.0	NS	7 (50%)	0	7 (50%)	
Hainsworth (46)	33[c]	No	135	CDDP 60 d2 E 100 d1–3	NS	12 (36%)	12 (36%)	72%	
Hainsworth (47)	82 50 eval	No	225	CBDA AUC 6.0	NS	22 (44%)	1 (2%)	23 (46%)	
Gelmon (48)	16	No	100–140	CDDP 60	NS	8 (50%)	1 (6%)	9 (56%)	
Giaccone (52)	62 50 eval	No	100–250	CBDA 300–400 mg/m²	NS	5 (10%)	1 (2%)	6 (12%)	

[a] 18 pts with cycles q4w, 26 pat with cycles q3w.
[b] Cycles q2w.
[c] After two cycles pat received RT 60 Gy with concomitant P 5 mg/m² E 25 mg/m² d1-5+d8-12, T 135 d1.
eval = evaluable.

Table 2b Phase III Studies

Reference	Pts	Prior Rx	Schedule mg/m^2	Adeno/squamous/ other	RR	Notes
Bonomi (44)	560	No	T 250 (24 h) + G-CSF, P 75 IV d1 vs. 135 (24 h), P 75 IV d 1 vs. E 100 IV d 1–3, P 75 IV d 1	NS	32% 26% 12%	Trend for TC or TCG, not significant
Giaccone (43)	251 159 ev	No	P 80 d 1, Teniposide 100 d 1,3,5 vs. P 80 d 1, T 175 (3-h) d 1	52/25/23	33%	5 toxic deaths 3 CR

Abbreviations: T = Taxol; P = cisplatin; E = etoposide.

Table 2bc Paclitaxel (Taxol) in NSCLC, Stage III Only

Reference	Pts	Adeno/squamous others %	Stage	CT	RT	Resection	RR
Adelstein (34)	16 eval	31/21/48	III (not T3N0)	CDDP 20 d 1–4 (24 h) + Taxol 175 d 1 (24 h) × 2 cycles	1.5 Gy bid (30 Gy) × 2 cycles	12 pat	63% PR
Siddiqui (41)	16	NS	III (NS)	Taxol 80–120 (3 h) d 1 E 40 d 2–5 IV CBDA AUC 4.0 d 1	NS	9 pat	68%
Choy (42)	33	NS	Unresect-able IIIA and IIIB	Taxol 60 mg/m^2 weekly for 6 weeks	60 Gy	No	2 CR (7%), 23 PR (79%)

Main toxicity was hematological but fluid retention was documented in most patients with increasing numbers of cycles. In most of these patients prolonged steroid therapy, a prerequisite in paclitaxel (Taxol) treatment, was not given (Table 3).

Combination of docetaxel (Taxotere) with platinum analogs was studied at different dose levels (22,26,32,50,51) with an OR of 30% to 46%. More pronounced myelotoxicity was found in the combination than in the single-agent docetaxel (Taxotere). Three more studies (27,30,45) investigated the combination of docetaxel (Taxotere) with vinorelbine (Navelbine®). The response rate was 23% to 47% (Table 4).

Phase II Results of Paclitaxel (Taxol) in SCLC

Two studies were conducted with paclitaxel 250 mg/m^2 in non-pretreated patients with extensive disease SCLC (1,2). A PR rate of 53% (1) resp. 68% (2) was reported with no CRs. Even as a second-line therapy, activity was found in 35% (36) of the patients; three of the patients were limited disease and 13 extensive disease stage (Table 5a).

The combination chosen with docetaxel (Taxotere) was cisplatin and etoposide in two small series (5,6) with a high CR rate of 56% in a small number of nine patients treated with docetaxel (Taxotere) 135 to 200 mg/m^2 IV over 3 h in combination with etoposide and cisplatinum. All nine patients responded with a PR or CR. These excellent results were confirmed in a similar study of 28 patients (4) with an overall response of 93% including 30% CRs. The patient stage was LD in 13 and ED in 15 patients. Again paclitaxel (Taxol) was given at a high dose of even 200 mg/m^2 as a 1-h infusion (Table 6).

Phase II Results of Docetaxel in SCLC

A study by Smyth et al. (3) has investigated docetaxel (Taxotere) in pretreated small-cell lung cancer patients. There were seven PRs in a total of 28 patients (25% PR) with no CR showing clear evidence for activity of docetaxel (Taxotere) in even pretreated small-cell lung cancer patients (Table 7b).

Table 3 NSCLC, Single-Agent Docetaxel (Taxotere)

Reference	Pts	Prior Rx	Dose mg/m²	Adeno/squamous/ other (%)	PR	CR	Notes
Cerny (12)	35	10 RT	100	44/29/27	7 (20%)	1 (3%)	Median surv 11 mo
Francis (13)	29	No	100	76/14/10	11 (38%)	0	
Burris (14)	14	No	100	NS	3 (21%)	0	
Fossella (15)	39	No	100	65/21/14	13 (33%)	0	
Watanabe (16)	68	No	60	63/30/7	12 (18%)	0	
Miller (17)	20	No	75	70/15/15	5 (25%)	0	
Burris (14)	15	Yes	100	NS	3 (20%)	0	
Fossella (18)	42	Yes	100	26/?/?	9 (21%)	0	
Mattson (23)	57[a]	43 No, 14 Yes	100	NS	14 (31%)	0	
Robinet (29)	53	5 RT	100	24/70/6	16 (30%)	0	
Robinet (31)	21[b]	Yes	100	43/52/5	4 (26%)	0	
Kath (33)	25	20 No, 5 Yes	100	10/10/5	4 (17%)	0	

RT = Radiotherapy.
[a]45 Pts evaluable for response.
[b]15 Pts evaluable for response.

Table 4 NSCLC, Docetaxel (Taxotere) Combinations

Reference	Pat	Previous Rx	Taxotere mg/m²	Other mg/m²	Adeno/squamous/other (%)	PR	CR	PR+CR
Bérille (22)	47[a]	No	75	CDDP 75	49/32/19	—	—	30%
	51[b]	No	75	CDDP 100	43/45/12	—	—	30%
Viallet (26)	41[c]	No	100	CDDP 100/VNR 30	75/?/?	17 (42%)	1 (2%)	18 (44%)
Kourousis (27)	32[d]	No	100	VNR 25	51/49/0	13 (41%)	2 (6%)	15 (47%)
Trillet-Lenoir (30)	34	No	75	VNR 20	41/28/31	9 (27%)	0	9 (27%)
Androulakis (32)	19[d]	No	100	CDDP 80	38/46/16	8 (42%)	0	8 (42%)
Monnier (45)	26	No	75	VNR 20	35/31/34	6 (23%)	0	6 (23%)
Cole, JT (50)	25	No	75	CDDP 75-100	NS	NS	NS	10 (46%)
Monnier (51)	51	No	75	CDDP 100	43/45/12	14 (28%)	1 (2%)	15 (30%)

[a]Cycles q3w.
[b]3 Cycles q3w then q6w.
[c]CDDP/VNR alternated to docetaxel.
[d]With G-CSF support.

Table 5a SCLC, Single-Agent Paclitaxel (Taxol)

Reference	Pts	LD/ED	Prior Rx	Dose mg/m^2	PR (%)	CR (%)
Ettinger (1)	34ED	No	250	17 (53%)	0	
Kirschling (2)	37	ED	No	250	25 (68%)	0
Smit (36)	16	3 LD	Yes	150–200	5 (35%)	0
	(14 eval)	13 ED				

[a]Only 2 cycles with Taxol.

Table 5b SCLC, Docetaxel (Taxotere), Single Agent

Reference	Pts	LD/ED	Prior Rx	Taxotere dose	PR (%)	CR (%)
Smyth (3)	28	LD and ED	27 yes	100 mg/m^2	7 (25%)	0

Table 6 SCLC, Paclitaxel (Taxol) Combinations

Reference	Combinations	Pts	Stage LD/ED	Prior Rx	PR (%)	CR (%)
Bunn (5)[a]	PET[b]	9	NS	No	4 (44%)	5 (56%)
Levitan (6)[a]	PET	8	ED	No	6 (75%)	1 (13%)
Georgiadis (7)[a]	PT[c]	6	ED	No	4 (66%)	0
Hainsworth (4)	CET[d]	28	LD 13 ED 15	No	17 (63%)	8 (30%)

P = cisplatin; E = etoposide; T = paclitaxel; C = carboplatin.
[a]Phase I studies.
[b]T 135–200 mg/m^2 IV 3 h, E 80 d 1 IV and 160 d$_{2-3}$ PO mg/m^2, P 80 d 1 IV.
[c]T in 96-h infusion.
[d]T 200 mg/m^2 (1-h inf), C AUC 6.0, E 75 mg d 1–10 PO q21d. LD received local RT (45 Gy).

Toxicity of Paclitaxel (Taxol)

Paclitaxel's (Taxol) main toxicity is predictable leukopenia, rather short lasting and usually not associated with infection. The main non-hematological toxicity is peripheral neurotoxicity which depends on cumulative dose but in some patients occurs even after one cycle. An unusual toxicity is myalgia which might become very disturbing and does not respond well to analgesics. Anaphylactic reactions are well prevented by steroid premedication, and alopecia is seen in almost all patients whereas mucositis is less often reported and rather mild.

Toxicity of Docetaxel (Taxotere)

As with paclitaxel (Taxol) main toxicity for docetaxel (Taxotere) is short-lasting leukopenia usually not associated with infections. Non-hematological main toxicity is peripheral neurotoxicity, which is cumulative. Myalgia is not a major problem but edema and pleural infusions is a typical cumulative toxicity in up to half of patients. It is not yet clear if this might be due to the lack of steroid premedication as it is mandatory for paclitaxel (Taxol). Mild to moderate hypersensitivity reactions have been found in 10% to 20% of patients. Alopecia is seen in almost all patients, and some patients also had nail changes with continuing therapy.

CONCLUSIONS

Overall, paclitaxel (Taxol) and docetaxel (Taxotere) have introduced themselves as major drugs of the 1990s in treatment of NSCLC and SCLC. They are active in pretreated and nonpretreated patients, and their activity might be greatly enhanced in combination with other standard drugs in treatment of lung cancer. Toxicity is manageable for both drugs, and activity is comparable for paclitaxel (Taxol) and docetaxel (Taxotere). The full potential of these powerful drugs has yet to be defined in further studies addressing the question of maximal activity and minimal toxicity in order to optimize future treatment strategies in curative and palliative attempts.

Table 7a Toxicity: Paclitaxel (Taxol)

Reference	Pts	Paclitaxel dose mg/m^2	Combinations	Neurotoxicity (%) (grade 1-3)	Mucositis (%)	Leukopenia (%)	Others (%)
(10, 11)	105	200–225/3 h	—	20 (56)	Rare	80	4% toxic deaths
(1, 8, 9)	83	250/24 h	—	15 (20)	2–6%	60–80	
(7, 25, 35, 49)	158	135–200	CDDP	6 (50)	Rare-17%	40–60	3–6 (5%) nephrotoxicity Myalgia (grade 2–3) (10–15%)
(4, 19, 24, 28, 37, 38, 47)	279	120–225	CBDA	5 (30)	Rare	40–80	Myalgia (10–15%) (grade 2–3)

Generally: Mucositis (grade <3) 1–30%; myalgia in (grade 2–3) 30–50%; anorexia (grade 1–3) 20–30%; alopecia, 80–100%.

Table 7b Toxicity: Docetaxel (Taxotere)

Reference	Pts	Docetaxel dose mg/m^2	Combinations	Neurotoxicity (%) (grade 1–3)	Mucositis (%)	Leukopenia (%)	Others (%) (grade 1–3)
(12, 13, 15, 16, 17, 23, 29)	387	100	—	20–40	Rare	40–90	Diarrhea 3–20 Pleural effusion 20–40 Edema 40–60
(22, 26, 50)	165	75–100	CCDP	17–40	Rare	40–90	Diarrhea 13–40
(27, 30, 45)	101	75–100	VNR	18–30	10–40	34–80	Edema 5–35

Generally: Hypersensitivity reactions, 10–20% (mild to moderate); alopecia, 80–90%; skin reactions, 30–60% (mild to moderate).

REFERENCES

1. Ettinger DS, Finkelstein DM, Sarma DM, et al. Phase II study of paclitaxel in patients with extensive disease small cell lung cancer. An Eastern Cooperative Oncology Group Study. J Clin Oncol 1995; 13: 1430–1435.
2. Kirschling RJ, Jung SH, Jett JR, North Central Cancer Treatment Group. A Phase II trial of Taxol and G-CSF in previously untreated patients with extensive-stage small cell lung cancer (SCLC). Proc Am Soc Clin Oncol 1994; 13:326. Abstract.
3. Smyth JF, Smith IE, Sessa C, et al. Activity of docetaxel in small cell lung cancer. Eur J Cancer 1994; 30A:1058–1060.
4. Hainsworth JD, Stroup SL, Gray JR, et al. Paclitaxel (one hour infusion), carboplatin and extended schedule etoposide in small cell lung cancer: a second generation phase II study. Proc ASCO 1996; 15:400. Abstract.
5. Bunn PA Jr, Kelly K. A phase I study of cisplatin, etoposide and paclitaxel in small cell lung cancer. A University of Colorado Cancer Center Study. Semin Oncol 1995; 22(suppl 2):54–58.
6. Levitan N, McKenney J, Tahsildar H, Ettinger D. Results of a Phase I dose escalation trial of paclitaxel, etoposide and cisplatin followed by filgrastim in the treatment of patients with extensive stage small cell lung cancer. Proc ASCO 1995; 14:379. Abstract.
7. Georgiadis MS, Brown JE, Schuler BS, et al. Phase I study of a four day continuous infusion of paclitaxel followed by cisplatin in patients with advanced lung cancer. Proc ASCO 1995; 14:353. Abstract.
8. Chang AY, Kim K, Glick J, Anderson T. A Phase II study of taxol, merbarone, and piroxantrone in Stage IV non-small cell lung cancer: the Eastern Cooperative Oncology Group Results. J Natl Cancer Inst 1993; 85(5):388–394.
9. Murphy WK, Fossella FV, Winn RJ, et al. Phase II study of taxol in patients with untreated advanced non-small cell lung cancer. J Natl Cancer Inst 1993; 85(5):384–387.
10. Gatzemeier U, Heckmayr M, Neuhauss R, et al. Phase II study with paclitaxel for the treatment of advanced inoperable non-small cell lung cancer. Lung Cancer 1995; 12(suppl 2):S101–S106.
11. Hainsworth JD, Hopkins L, Thomas M, et al. Taxol administered by one hour infusion: preliminary results of a phase I/II study comparing two dose schedules. Lung Cancer 1994; 11(suppl 11):96. Abstract.

12. Cerny T, Kaplan S, Pavlidis N, et al. Docetaxel (Taxotere) is active in non-small cell lung cancer: A phase II trial of the EORTC early clinical trials group (LCTG). Br J Cancer 1994; 70:384–387.
13. Francis PA, Riga JR, Kris MG, et al. Phase II trial of docetaxel in patients with Stage III and IV non-small cell lung cancer. J Clin Oncol 1994; 12:1232–1237.
14. Burris H, Eckardt J, Fields S, et al. Phase II trials of taxotere in patients with non-small cell lung cancer. Proc Am Soc Clin Oncol 1993; 12:335. Abstract.
15. Fossella FV, Lee JS, Murphy WK, et al. Phase II study of docetaxel for recurrent or metastatic non-small cell lung cancer. J Clin Oncol 1994; 12:1238–1244.
16. Watanabe K, Yokoyama A, Furuse K, et al. Phase II trial of docetaxel in previously untreated non-small cell lung cancer (NSCLC). Proc Am Soc Clin Oncol 1994; 13:331. Abstract.
17. Miller VA, Rigas R, Kile MG, et al. Phase II trial of docetaxel given at a dose of 75 mg/m^2 with prednisone premedication in non-small cell lung cancer (NSCLC). Proc Am Soc Clin Oncol 1994; 13:364. Abstract.
18. Fossella FV, Lee JS, Shin DM, et al. Phase II study of docetaxel for advanced or metastatic platinum-refractory non-small cell lung cancer. J Clin Oncol 1995; 13:645–651.
19. Langer CJ, Leighton JC, Comis RL, et al. Paclitaxel and carboplatin in combination in the treatment of advanced non-small cell lung cancer: a phase II toxicity, response and survival analysis. J Clin Oncol 1995; 13(8):1860–1870.
20. Belani CP, Aisner J, Hiponia D, Engstrom C. Paclitaxel and carboplatin with and without filgrastim support in patients with metastatic non-small cell lung cancer. Semin Oncol 1995; 22(suppl 9):7–12.
21. Johnson DH, Paul DM, Hande KR, et al. Paclitaxel (taxol) plus carboplatin for advanced lung cancer: preliminary results of a Vanderbilt University phase II trial-LUN-46. Sem Oncol 1995; 22(suppl 9): 30–33.
22. Bérille J, Le Chevalier T, Zalcberg JR, et al. Overview on Taxotere-cisplatin (TXT-CDDP) combination in non-small cell cancer. Ann Oncol 1996; 7(suppl 5):90. Abstract.
23. Mattson K, Le Chevalier T, Stupp R, et al. Preliminary report of a phase II study of docetaxel (taxotere) in locally advanced or metastatic non-small cell lung cancer (NSCLC). Ann Oncol 1996; 7(suppl 5):90. Abstract.

24. Kosmidis P, Mylonakis N, Fountzilas G, et al. Phase II study of paclitaxel and carboplatin in inoperable non-small cell lung cancer (NSCLC). Ann Oncol 1996; 7(suppl 5):90. Abstract.

25. Von Pawel G, Wagner H, Niederle N, et al. Phase II study of paclitaxel and cisplatin in patients with non-small cell lung cancer (NSCLC). Ann Oncol 1996; 7(suppl 5):91. Abstract.

26. Viallet J, Laberge F, Martins H, et al. A Phase II trial of docetaxel alternating with cisplatin and vinorelbine in non-small cell lung cancer. Ann Oncol 1996; 7(suppl 5):93. Abstract.

27. Kourousis C, Kakolyris S, Androulakis N, et al. First line treatment of non-small cell lung carcinoma (NSCLC) with docetaxel and vinorelbine: a phase II study. Proc ASCO 1996; 15:405. Abstract.

28. Steppert C, Bültzingslöwen F, Weiss J, et al. Polychemotherapy with carboplatin (CBDA) and paclitaxel in advanced NSCLC—a phase II study. Ann Oncol 1996; 7(suppl 5):93. Abstract.

29. Robinet G, Thomas P, Kleisbauer JP, et al. Phase II study of docetaxel in metastatic non-small cell lung cancer (NSCLC): prevention of fluid retention with 5 days steroid and continuous flavonoids. Ann Oncol 1996; 7(suppl 5):94. Abstract.

30. Trillet-Lenoir V, Monnier A, Douillard JY, et al. Interim results of a phase II study of docetaxel (Taxotere) and vinorelbine in chemotherapy naive patients with advanced non-small cell lung carcinoma (NSCLC). Ann Oncol 1996; 7(suppl 5):95. Abstract.

31. Robinet G, Thomas P, Perol M, et al. Phase II study of taxotere in advanced or metastatic non-small cell lung cancer (NSCLC) previously treated with platinum. Ann Oncol 1996; 7(suppl 5):96. Abstract.

32. Androulakis N, Kourousis C, Kakolyris S. First line treatment of non-small cell lung cancer with docetaxel and cis-platin: preliminary results of a phase II study. Ann Oncol 1996; 7(suppl 5):98. Abstract.

33. Kath R, Blumenstengel K, Fricke HJ, et al. Preliminary report of chemotherapy results with docetaxel in advanced non-small cell lung cancer (NSCLC). Ann Oncol 1996; 7(suppl 5):100. Abstract.

34. Adelstein DJ, Rice TW, Becker M, et al. Accelerated fractionation (AFR), concurrent cisplatin/paclitaxel chemotherapy and surgery for stage III non-small cell lung cancer: preliminary toxicity. Proc ASCO 1996; 15:391. Abstract.

35. Sorensen JB, Wederwang K, Bjarnoe H, et al. Biweekly paclitaxel and cisplatin for nonresectable non-small cell lung cancer (NSCLC). Proc ASCO 1996; 15:394. Abstract.

36. Smit EF, Kloosterziel C, Groen HJM, Postmus PE. A Phase II study of paclitaxel in heavily pretreated patients with small cell lung cancer (SCLC). ASCO 1996; 15:394. Abstract.
37. Langer C, Kaplan R, Rosvold E, et al. Paclitaxel by 1 hour infusion combined with carboplatin in advanced non-small cell lung carcinoma (NSCLC): a phase II study. ASCO 1996; 15:396. Abstract.
38. Schütte W, Bork I, Sucker S, Schädlich ST. Phase II trial of paclitaxel and carboplatin as firstline treatment in advanced non-small cell lung cancer (NSCLC). ASCO 1996; 15:398. Abstract.
39. Roa V, Conner A, Mitchell RB. Carboplatin and paclitaxel for advanced non-small cell lung cancer in previously treated patients. ASCO 1996; 15:403. Abstract.
40. Roa V, Conner A, Mitchell RB. Carboplatin and paclitaxel for chemotherapy naive patients with advanced non-small cell lung cancer. ASCO 1996; 15:404. Abstract.
41. Siddiqui S, Bonomi P, Faber LP, et al. Phase I-II trial of escalating doses of paclitaxel, carboplatin, etoposide and simultaneous thoracic radiation ± pulmonary resection in stage III non-small cell lung cancer. ASCO 1996; 15:405. Abstract.
42. Choy H, Akerley W, Safran H, et al. Phase II trial of weekly paclitaxel and concurrent radiation therapy for locally advanced non-small cell lung cancer. ASCO 1996; 15:371. Abstract.
43. Giaccone G, Splinter T, Postmus P, et al. Paclitaxel-cisplatin versus Teniposide-cisplatin in advanced non-small cell lung cancer (NSCLC). ASCO 1996; 15:373. Abstract.
44. Bonomi P, Kim K, Chang A, Johnson D. Phase III trial comparing etoposide cisplatin versus taxol with cisplatin-G-CFS versus taxol cisplatin in advanced non-small cell lung cancer. An Eastern Cooperative Oncology Group (ECOG) trial. ASCO 1996; 15:382. Abstract.
45. Monnier A, Riviere A, Douillard JY, et al. Phase II study of docetaxel (Taxotere) and vinorelbine in chemotherapy naive patients with advanced non-small cell lung carcinoma (NSCLC). ASCO 1996; 15:378. Abstract.
46. Hainsworth JD, Stroup SL, Gray JR, et al. Paclitaxel (1-hour infusion), cisplatin, etoposide and radiation therapy in locally advanced, unresectable non-small cell lung cancer (NSCLC). ASCO 1996; 15:379. Abstract.
47. Hainsworth JD, Thompson DS, Urba WJ, et al. One hour paclitaxel plus carboplatin in advanced non-small cell lung cancer (NSCLC).

Preliminary results of a multi-institutional phase II study. Proc ASCO 1996; 15:379. Abstract.

48. Gelmon KA, Mrray N, Melosky B, et al. Phase I-II study of biweekly paclitaxel (taxol) and cisplatin in non-small cell lung cancer (NSCLC). ASCO 1996; 15:405. Abstract.

49. Belli L, Le Chevalier T, Gottfried M, et al. Phase I-II trial of paclitaxel and cisplatin in previously untreated advanced non-small cell lung cancer (NSCLC). ASCO 1995; 14:350. Abstract.

50. Cole JT, Gralla RJ, Marques CB, Rittenberg CN. Phase I-II study of cisplatin and docetaxel in non-small cell lung cancer (NSCLC). ASCO 1995; 14:357. Abstract.

51. Monnier A, Douillard JY, Belli L, et al. Interim analysis of a phase II study of docetaxel and cisplatin in advanced non-small cell lung cancer. SOMPS 1996; 77.

52. Giaccone G, Huizing M, Postmus P, et al. Dose finding and sequencing study of paclitaxel and carboplatin in non-small cell lung cancer. Semin Oncol 1995; 22(suppl 9):78–82.

5

Paclitaxel in the Treatment of Small-Cell Lung Cancer

North American Experience

David S. Ettinger
The Johns Hopkins Oncology Center, Baltimore, Maryland

INTRODUCTION

A number of drugs are active as single agents in the treatment of small-cell lung cancer (SCLC) (1). With so many active drugs, many different effective combination chemotherapeutic regimens have been developed to treat SCLC. Unfortunately, despite these effective therapies, most patients with SCLC will eventually die of their disease. The identification of new drugs with significant activity against lung cancer is needed. One such new drug is paclitaxel (Taxol; Bristol-Myers Squibb Co., Princeton, NJ) (2).

The results of the initial two Phase II studies of paclitaxel conducted by both the Eastern Cooperative Oncology Group (ECOG) (3) and North Central Cancer Treatment Group (NCCTG) (4,5) as well as three studies utilizing paclitaxel in combination chemotherapeutic regimens (6–10) to treat previously untreated SCLC patients will be reported.

SINGLE-AGENT TREATMENT: ECOG STUDY

This Phase II study was activated by ECOG in October 1990 and closed in October 1991. Thirty-six patients were registered, with 34 patients evaluable for toxicity and 32 patients evaluable for response. Of the 34 patients receiving paclitaxel, 24 received salvage chemotherapy (VP-16 + cisplatin). Table 1 lists patient and disease characteristics of the 34 evaluable patients.

Patients and Methods

Patients with histologically or cytologically confirmed SCLC with extensive-stage disease, having an ECOG performance status of 0, 1, or 2; and adequate bone marrow (WBC $\geq$ 4,000/μL and platelet count $\geq$ 100,000/μL), liver (bilirubin $\leq$ 2.0 mg/dL), and kidney (creatinine $\leq$ 1.5 mg/dL and blood urea nitrogen level $\leq$ 25 mg/dL), function with measurable disease, no prior chemotherapy, no brain metastases, and no recent cardiac disease, were eligible. Patients were ineligible for the study if they had prior irradiation to any sites of disease.

Before entry into the study all patients underwent a staging evaluation consisting of a complete history and physical examination; complete blood cell count (CBC); routine blood chemistries; chest roentgenogram; computer tomographic (CT) scan of chest, abdomen, and brain; and bone scan. A bone marrow aspiration and biopsy and fiberoptic bronchoscopy were also performed.

During cycle 1, patients were evaluated weekly, and a CBC count was performed routinely. At 3-week intervals, just before each cycle of drug administration, response was assessed by obtaining serum chemistries, a chest roentgenogram, and tumor measurements, in addition to the CBC count. Additional CBC counts were performed as clinically indicated. All positive tests were to be repeated before the fifth chemotherapy cycle and at the time clinical complete response (CR) was diagnosed. Complete responders were monitored every 3 months with a CBC count, serum chemistries, CT scan of the chest and abdomen, and bone scan. Standard ECOG criteria for solid tumor response were used (11).

Table 1 Patient and Disease Characteristics

	No. of patients	%
Patients	36	
Evaluable for toxicity	34	
Evaluable for response	32	
Sex		
Male	21	62
Female	13	38
Race (white)	33	97
Age, years		
Median	63	
Range	40–78	
Initial performance status		
0	9	26
1	19	
2	6	18
Prior weight loss (%)		
None	13	38
<5	10	29
5–10	6	18
>10	5	15
Sites of distant metastases		
Ipsilateral lung	22	65
Contralateral lung	3	9
Mediastinum	24	71
Pleura	7	21
Scalene lymph node	7	21
Liver	22	65
Bone marrow	9	26
Bone	7	21
Subcutaneous	1	3
Other	10	29
No. of distant metastases		
1	3	9
2	6	18
3	10	29
4	10	29
5	3	9
≥6	2	6

(continued)

Table 1 Continued

	No. of patients	%
Response		
CR	0	0
PR	11	34
SD	6	19
Progression	15	47
Grade 4 and 5 toxicity		
Lcukopenia	19	56
Pulmonary	3	9
Hepatic	2	6
Cardiac	1	3
Thrombocytopenia	1	3
Stomatitis	1	3
Allergic reaction	1	3
Sepsis (lethal)	1	3

Treatment

Patients with extensive-disease SCLC received paclitaxel 250 mg/m^2 administered intravenously over 24 h every 3 weeks. Because of a limited drug supply at the time this study was activated, patients received a maximum of four doses of paclitaxel as induction therapy. Patients with disease progression after one cycle of therapy or stable disease (SD) after two cycles or who achieved a partial response (PR) only after four cycles of paclitaxel received salvage chemotherapy that consisted of VP-16 120 mg/m^2 intravenously over 45 min on days 1, 2, and 3, and cisplatin 60 mg/m^2 intravenously as a short infusion on day 1. Cycles were repeated every 3 weeks. Patients who attained a CR were to receive a minimum of four cycles of chemotherapy. Prophylactic whole-brain irradiation (25 Gy in 10 fractions over 2 weeks) was to be given to patients who achieved a CR, beginning 1 week after completion of induction therapy.

 If progression occurred after induction therapy had been completed in patients who attained a CR, the patients were to receive salvage chemotherapy. Patients with disease progression after one cycle of salvage chemotherapy or with SD after two cycles were removed from study. Those who achieved only a PR after salvage chemotherapy continued therapy until progression of disease and were then removed from study. Patients who achieved a CR on salvage chemotherapy received six to eight cycles of therapy and then no maintenance chemotherapy. If a CR was obtained on salvage chemotherapy, prophylactic whole-brain irradiation was to be given if the patient had not already received it.

Drug doses were modified for hematological toxicity. Dose modifications were also made for renal or hepatic dysfunction, mucositis, and auditory, neurological, or cardiac toxicity.

Toxicity

Treatment complications were reported according to ECOG standard criteria by degree (none, mild, moderate, severe, life-threatening, or lethal), by type (gastrointestinal, vomiting, etc.), and by cause. Table 2 lists the incidence of severe and life-threatening complications from the therapy with paclitaxel. ECOG grade 4 hematological toxicity occurred in 19 patients (56%) with leukopenia and one patient (3%) with thrombocytopenia while receiving paclitaxel. Nonhematological life-threatening toxicities that occurred during induction therapy, due to paclitaxel, consisted of the following:

1. Pulmonary, three patients (9%). Specifically, one patient experienced pulmonary edema during day 2 of cycle 1; another patient developed respiratory failure on day 11 of cycle 2 and was placed on a ventilator and then home oxygen; and a third patient experienced wheezing and shortness of breath during day 2 of cycle 1.
2. Hepatic, two patients (6%) with known liver metastases developed elevated liver function tests.
3. Cardiac, one patient (3%) developed an acute myocardial infarction during day 16 of cycle 3.
4. Metabolic, one patient (3%) developed hypocalcemia during day 3 of cycle 1.

Table 2   Incidence of Severe and Life-Threatening
Complications

Complication	Paclitaxel	
	Severe	Life-threatening
Leukopenia	4	19
Thrombocytopenia	—	1
Anemia	—	—
Infection	4	—
Nausea	1	—
Vomiting	—	—
Diarrhea	1	—
Stomatitis	1	1
Hepatic	5	2
Pulmonary	1	3
Cardiac	2	1
Hypertension	—	—
Neuroclinical	1	—
Neuromotor	1	—
Metabolic	1	1
Allergy	1	1
Dysphagia	1	—

5. Stomatitis, one patient (3%) experienced reddening and swelling in the mouth during day 9 of cycle 1.
6. Allergy, one patient (3%) developed anaphylaxis during day 2 of cycle 1.

Response

Among 34 patients who could be analyzed while on induction, two were unevaluable because of inadequate response documentation. All available patients had at least one two-dimensional measurable lesion. On induction therapy, there were no CRs; however, there were 11 PRs (34%). Six patients had SD. In three of these six, there was a > 50% tumor shrinkage; however, there were no 4-week follow-up measurements, partly because the patients received salvage chemotherapy 3 weeks after their last dose of paclitaxel. Therefore, three patients were not considered as having had a PR since, by definition, such a response must last at least 4 weeks.

Response duration was measured from the time a response was documented to the time of relapse or patient last known to be in response (censored). For the 11 patients who responded to paclitaxel, the median response duration was 12 weeks, with a range of 5 to 33 weeks. The response duration may be falsely low because responding patients who received four cycles of paclitaxel, by study design, had to be crossed over to salvage therapy when, in fact, they might have been still responding to paclitaxel.

Survival

Overall survival was measured from the date of registration to date of death due to any cause or date last known to be alive (censored). Of 34 assessable patients, one was censored for this analysis, because the patient moved and was lost for follow-up evaluation. The estimated median survival time was 43 weeks.

NCCTG STUDY

The NCCTG conducted a trial similar to the ECOG study to confirm the activity of paclitaxel in patients with extensive-stage SCLC. Forty-three patients were entered into the study, with 37 patients evaluable for response and toxicity. Patients with disease progression or stable disease after six cycles of paclitaxel received VP-16 + cisplatin. Table 3 lists patients and disease characteristics of the 37 evaluable patients.

Patients and Methods

Patient eligibility criteria were similar to that in the ECOG study, as was the treatment evaluation. Tumor responses were defined as CR or PR in patients with measurable disease and as CR or regression in those with assessable disease, using the previously described criteria of the NCCTG (12,13).

Table 3 Patient and Disease Characteristics

Characteristic	No. of patients	%
Patients	43	
Evaluable for toxicity	37	
Evaluable for response	32	
Sex		
Male	27	63
Female	16	37
Age, years		
Median	66	
Range	34–83	
Initial performance status		
0, 1, or 2	37	
Response		
CR	0	0
PR	15	40.5
Major response	10	27
SD	?	
Progression	?	
Grade 4 toxicity (n=37)		
Leukopenia	(19% of course)	
Stomatitis	1	
Diarrhea	1	
Infection	1	
Pulmonary	1	

Treatment

Patients received paclitaxel 250 mg/m^2 by a 24-h infusion day 1 administered every 21 days. In this study granulocyte-colony stimulating factor (G-CSF) 5 μg/kg was administered subcutaneously on days 2 to 15 every 3 weeks. The salvage chemotherapy consisted of both etoposide 100 mg/m^2 intravenously and cisplatin 30 mg/m^2 intravenously for 3 consecutive days every 3 to 4 weeks.

Drug doses were modified for hematological toxicity as well as for mucositis. Drug therapy was discontinued in patients experiencing grade 3 or greater toxicities: cardiac, allergic reactions, and neuropathies.

Toxicity

Preliminary toxicity data are available for 37 patients. The primary toxicity observed has been myelosuppression. Grade 4 leukopenia occurred with 19% of treatment courses. There has been no significant thrombocytopenia. Other grade 4 toxicities encountered thus far have consisted of one case each of stomatitis, diarrhea, infection, and pulmonary toxicity.

Response

Thirty-seven patients were evaluable for response. There were no CRs and 15 PRs. Ten additional patients with assessable disease had a major response. The overall response rate was 67.5%.

Survival

The median survival duration was 29 weeks.

COMBINATION CHEMOTHERAPY: UNIVERSITY OF COLORADO CANCER CENTER STUDY

Bunn et al. (6,7) at the University of Colorado Cancer Center performed a dose escalation study in untreated extensive-stage SCLC patients utilizing paclitaxel 135 to 175 mg/m^2 as a 3-h infusion; etoposide 50 to 80 mg/m^2 IV day 1; 100 to 160 mg/m^2 PO days 2 and 3 every 3 weeks until disease progression or for 6 cycles. G-CSF was given starting on cycle 2 only in case of grade 4 neutropenia during cycle 1 or if the cycle had to be prolonged for > 4 weeks because of persistent neutropenia.

At the time of their reports, 16 patients had been entered on study at three different dose levels (Table 4). The overall response rate was 100% (25% CR + 75% PR). Thirteen of 16 patients had

Table 4 Study Doses, Response, and Toxicity

Level (# pts)	Drugs (mg/m^2)			Response		Grade 4 toxicities	
	Paclitaxel	Cisplatin	Etoposide	CR	PR	Granulo-cytopenia	Platelets
1 (5)	135	80	50 IV day 1 100 PO day 2, 3	2/3	1/3	2/5	0/5
2 (5)	135	80	80 IV day 1 160 PO day 2, 3	1/3	2/3	5/5	1/5
3 (6)	175	80	80 IV day 1 160 PO day 2, 3	0/6	6/6	6/6	0/6

grade 4 neutropenia; however, only eight of 11 patients in dose levels 2 and 3 required G-CSF. Only one patient at dose level 3 developed febrile neutropenia. Nonhematological toxicities were mild. Patients were being entered on dose level 4 receiving paclitaxel 200 mg/m^2.

IRELAND CANCER CENTER STUDY

Levitan et al. (8) from the Ireland Cancer Center, University Hospitals of Cleveland, performed a dose-escalation study of paclitaxel 135-170-200 mg/m^2 (3-h infusion) and cisplatin 60 mg/m^2 on day 1 and etoposide 80 mg/m^2 IV on days 1 to 3 given to previously untreated extensive-stage SCLC patients every 21 days. G-CSF was administered at a dose of 5 μg/kg subcutaneously on days 5 to 14. Of the eight patients entered on study, one had achieved a CR and six had PRs for an overall response rate of 88%. No toxicity was seen in patients receiving paclitaxel 135 mg/m^2 along with cisplatin and etoposide; however, at the 170 mg/m^2 dose level, two patients experienced grade III and IV diarrhea, respectively, while one patient experienced grade III neutropenia (sepsis). Dose escalation was terminated at a paclitaxel dose of 170 mg/m^2.

SARAH CANNON CANCER CENTER STUDY

Hainsworth et al. (9) from the Sarah Cannon Cancer Center performed a study of paclitaxel 135 mg/m^2 administered as a 1-h infusion with carboplatin dosed at an AUC = 5 using the Calvert formula on day 1 and etoposide 50 mg PO alternating with 100 mg PO on days 1 to 10 in untreated patients with both limited-stage and extensive-stage SCLC. Patients with limited-stage SCLC received concurrent radiation therapy (4500 cGy/25 fractions) starting on their third cycle of chemotherapy. Twenty-nine patients received the therapy (13, limited-stage; 16, extensive-stage). Of the 22 patients evaluable for response, 10 achieved a CR (45%) and 11 achieved a PR (50%). Of the CRs, six patients had limited-stage while four patients had extensive-stage SCLC. At the time of the report, 15 patients were progression-free after a median of 8 months of follow-up. Grade 3/4 toxicities included leukopenia (18% of courses), thrombocytopenia (four patients), neutropenic fever (eight patients required hospitalization), and esophagitis during RT (four patients).

In a follow-up study (10), the dose of paclitaxel was escalated to 200 mg/m^2 as a 1-h infusion, while the carboplatin was dosed to AUC = 6. The etoposide dose and schedule was similar to the above schedule. Twenty-eight patients (13, limited-stage; 15, extensive-stage) were entered on study. Limited-stage patients received radiation therapy concurrently with chemotherapy beginning with the third cycle. Twenty-five of 27 evaluable patients (93%) had an objective response (eight CRs; 17 PRs). Fifty-four of limited-stage patients achieved a CR while 6% of extensive-stage patients achieved a PR. Grade 3/4 leukopenia occurred in 41% of courses of therapy. Eighteen patients were progression-free after a median of 6 months of follow-up.

OTHER LIMITED-STAGE STUDIES

Both RTOG and ECOG will be conducting a Phase II study of paclitaxel, etoposide, and cisplatin with radiotherapy for patients with limited-stage SCLC.

In the RTOG study, cycle 1 of chemotherapy will be given with concurrent twice daily radiotherapy (45 Gy in 30 fractions, 1.5 Gy per fraction; daily fractions to be separated by at least 6 hours. The chemotherapy will consist of paclitaxel 135 mg/m^2 as a 3-h infusion day 1, etoposide 60 mg/m^2 IV day 1; 80 mg/m^2 PO days 2, 3 and cisplatin 60 mg/m^2 IV day 1 every 3 weeks. Cycle 2–4 doses of chemotherapy will be the same as in cycle 1 except that the dose of paclitaxel will be increased to 175 mg/m^2. No G-CSF will be used until the radiotherapy is concluded.

In the ECOG study, cycle 1 and 2 will be given without radiotherapy which then will be given concurrently beginning with cycle 3 of the chemotherapy. The chemotherapy for all four cycles will be the same, consisting of paclitaxel 170 mg/m^2 as a 3-h infusion day 1, etoposide 60 mg/m^2 IV days 1 to 3, and cisplatin 60 mg/m^2 IV day 2. During the first two cycles all patients receive G-CSF 5 μg/kg subcutaneously days 5 to 14. Beginning with cycle 3 concurrent radiotherapy (63 Gy/35 fractions/7 weeks) will be given.

The SWOG has proposed a phase II trial of concurrent cisplatin, etoposide, vincristine, and radiotherapy followed by carboplatin/paclitaxel in patients with limited-stage SCLC. The induction therapy will consist of concurrent cisplatin 50 mg/m^2 IV d 1, 8, 29, 36, 57, 64; etoposide 50 mg/m^2 IV d 1–5, 29–33, 57–61; and vincristine 1.4 mg/m^2 (max 2.0 mg) IV d 15, 22, 43, 50 with thoracic radiotherapy 150 cGy bid, 5 day/wk for 3 weeks (total of 45 Gy). The consolidation therapy will consist of carboplatin dosed at an AUC of 6 and paclitaxel 200 mg/m^2 infused over 3 h every 21 days for four cycles.

ANOTHER EXTENSIVE-STAGE STUDY

In patients with extensive-stage SCLC, the CALGB is doing a three-arm study comparing cisplatin/topotecan to cisplatin/paclitaxel to paclitaxel/topotecan. The dose of cisplatin is 75 mg/m^2 IV day 1, topotecan 1 mg/m^2 as a 3-min infusion days 1 to 5, and paclitaxel 230 mg/m^2 as a 3-h infusion day 1. G-CSF is given in each of the arms. Each cycle is repeated every 3 weeks.

DISCUSSION

The results of the two Phase II studies conducted by ECOG and NCCTG demonstrate that paclitaxel is an active agent against SCLC. In both studies, paclitaxel 250 mg/m^2 was administered as a 24-h continuous infusion every 3 weeks. The three trials utilizing paclitaxel in combination with etoposide and either cisplatin or carboplatin demonstrate that these combinations have significant activity against SCLC.

Both ECOG and RTOG are to evaluate paclitaxel, etoposide, and cisplatin given concurrently with radiation therapy in patients with limited-stage SCLC.

There are a number of potential combination chemotherapeutic regimens that can contain paclitaxel to be studied in patients with SCLC. In addition, studies evaluating paclitaxel administered as a 3-h and 1-h infusion in combination with other agents are ongoing as well as studies evaluating the drug administered concurrently with radiation therapy.

REFERENCES

1. Feld R, Ginsberg RJ, Payne DG. Treatment of small cell lung cancer. In: Roth RA, Rickdeschel JC, Weisgenburger JH, eds. Thoracic Oncology. Philadelphia: Saunders, 1989:229–262.
2. Clinical brochure. Taxol (NSC-125973). Bethesda: National Cancer Institute, 1983.
3. Ettinger DS, Finkelstein DM, Sarma RP, Johnson DH. Phase II study of paclitaxel in patients with extensive-disease small cell lung cancer: An Eastern Cooperative Oncology Group study. J Clin Oncol 1995; 13:1430–1435.
4. Kirschling RJ, Jung SH, Jett JR. A phase II trial of Taxol and G-CSF in previously untreated patients with extensive stage small cell lung cancer. Proc Am Soc Clin Oncol 1994; 13:326. Abstract.
5. Jett JR, Kirschling RI, Jung SH, et al. A phase II study of paclitaxel and granulocyte colony-stimulating factor in previously untreated patients with extensive-stage small cell lung cancer: A study of the North Central Cancer Treatment Group. Semin Oncol 1995; 22(suppl 6): 75–77.

6. Bunn PA, Kelly KL. A phase I study of cisplatin, etoposide, and paclitaxel in small cell lung cancer: a University of Colorado Cancer Center
   Study. Semin Oncol 1995; 22(5:suppl 12):54–58.
7. Kelly K, Wood ME, Bunn PA. A phase I study of cisplatin, etoposide
   and paclitaxel (PET) in extensive-stage small cell lung cancer (SCLC).
   Proc Am Soc Clin Oncol 1995; 14:384. Abstract 1214.
8. Levitan N, McKenny J, Tahsildar H, Ettinger D. Results of a phase I
   dose escalation trial of paclitaxel, etoposide and cisplatin followed by
   filgrastim in treatment of patients with extensive-stage small cell lung
   cancer. Proc Am Soc Clin Oncol 1995; 14:379. Abstract 1177.
9. Hainsworth JD, McKay CE, Miller PS, Greco FA. Treatment of small
   cell lung cancer (SCLC) paclitaxel (one-hour infusion), carboplatin,
   and low dose etoposide. Proc Am Soc Clin Oncol 1995; 14:384. Abstract
   1197.
10. Hainsworth JD, Stroup SL, Gray JR, et al. Paclitaxel (1-hour infusion),
    carboplatin, and extended schedule etoposide in small cell lung cancer
    (SCLC): a second generation phase II study. Proc Am Soc Clin Oncol
    1996; 15:400. Abstract 1215.
11. Oken MM, Davis TE, Creech RH, et al. Toxicity and response criteria
    of the Eastern Cooperative Oncology Group. Am J Clin Oncol 1982;
    5:649–655.
12. Jett JR, Everson L, Therneau T, et al. Treatment of limited stage small
    cell lung cancer with cyclophosphamide, doxorubicin and vincristine
    with or without etoposide: a randomized trial of the North Central
    Cancer Treatment Group. J Clin Oncol 1990; 8:33–39.
13. Maksymiuk AW, Jett JR, Earle JD, et al. Sequencing and schedule
    effects of cisplatin plus etoposide in small cell lung cancer: Results of
    a North Central Cancer Treatment Group randomized clinical trial. J
    Clin Oncol 1994; 12:70–76.

6

Taxanes in Small-Cell Lung Cancer

European Experience

Nick Thatcher, M. Ranson, G. Jayson, and H. Anderson
Christie Hospital, Manchester, England

INTRODUCTION

In the European Community lung cancer accounts for 29% of all cancer deaths and 21% of all cancer cases in men. The mortality and incidence for women are lower—8% and 4%, respectively. The trend in mortality from lung cancer in the E.C. from 1970 to 1984 demonstrates a 10% to 15% increase among men every 5 years, except for the U.K., where there is a slight decrease. Among women the death rate has increased 15% to 30% every 5 years except in France, Greece, and Spain, where the increase has been somewhat less. Examination of the mortality patterns suggest that southern and eastern Europe will have the highest lung cancer rates at the beginning of the next century (1,2). Lung cancer will continue to be the major cancer problem in Europe for several decades to come unless effective tobacco control is instituted.

In the U.K. it is still the most frequently occurring cancer, accounting for one in seven new cases and on average one person dies every 15 min from the disease. Perhaps most worrying is the proportion of children who now smoke regularly. There has been an increase from 10% in 1992 to 12% in 1994, and, by the age of 15, one in four children is a regular smoker, girls having consistently higher rates of smoking than boys (3). Effective methods of discouraging young people from starting to smoke are essential, but there is still a need to develop much more effective treatment for the disease.

PROGNOSTIC GROUPS AND CHEMOTHERAPY

Several active agents have in the past been identified for the treatment of SCLC, and combination regimens have been developed based on this single-agent activity. The untreated survival is only a few weeks but has been extended about fivefold with the use of combination chemotherapy. Median survival times for the more favorable prognostic groups (good performance status, limited stage, etc.) are of the order of 14 to 16 months and 7 to 9 months in the poorer prognostic groups. Approximately one-third to one-half of patients fulfill the criteria for the better prognostic groups (4,5). The other, remaining patients with poorer prognostic features are usually considered for new drug studies. Nevertheless even with optimal chemotherapy < 10% of patients overall are alive at 5 years, indicating the urgent need for newer active agents (6).

For patients with better prognosis, research has recently concentrated on the use of newer drug combinations which have included platinum; intensification of treatment, especially with the advent of hemopoietic growth factor support; and hyperfractionated radiotherapy regimens in conjunction with chemotherapy. In the poorer-prognosis group of patients who are unlikely to tolerate or benefit from intensive treatment, including the elderly, patients with impaired performance status, extensive stage disease etc., palliation remains an important objective. However, this aim may not be realized by using what is considered by the nononcologist as "gentle, simple," e.g., oral etoposide chemotherapy.

Two recent randomized controlled trials have compared oral etoposide against intravenous combination chemotherapy in a population of poor prognosis patients. The larger British Medical Research Council study compared oral etoposide with intravenous combination chemotherapy—vincristine, doxorubicin, cyclophosphamide (VAC) in the majority of patients (IV etoposide and vincristine in the minority). A planned interim analysis by an Independent Data Monitoring Committee advised closure of the study when 339 patients of a planned intake of 450 had been randomized. The reasons for the decision were that palliation of cough, pain, anorexia, and breathlessness were inferior in the oral etoposide group together with worse hematological toxicity and an inferior survival. Median survivals were 132 days in the oral etoposide group and 183 days in the intravenous combination chemotherapy group ($p = .03$, hazard ratio .74) in this poor-prognosis group of patients. These results were counterintuitive and emphasized the need for appropriately constructed clinical trials to generate evidence based medicine (7). A similar although smaller study, again from the U.K., compared oral etoposide with intravenous chemotherapy cisplatin, etoposide alternating with the VAC regimen. Again there were worse survival and toxicity with single-agent oral etoposide (Ref. 8). Other approaches to palliation are clearly required for this group of patients with impaired performance status, and a convenient "easy-to-use" treatment can be suboptimal. Such patients could be considered for new drug trials.

PATIENT POPULATIONS FOR NEW DRUG EVALUATION

New drug investigation is, therefore, an extremely important issue in small-cell lung cancer (SCLC), where despite the tumor chemosensitivity there has been no substantial progress in treatment over the past few years. However, testing new drugs in these patients can give rise to difficult situations. Despite fairly short survival in the poor-prognosis group of patients current standard chemotherapy can provide effective palliation and some extension of survival. New drugs can, of course, be evaluated in patients who have failed on standard treatment, but potentially valuable agents may not be identified due to the presence of multidrug resistance.

One approach is to evaluate new agents with promising preclinical activity in patients with previously untreated extensive-stage disease providing that the patients who do not benefit from the new treatment are not subsequently compromised when standard chemotherapy is used for salvage (9,10). However, in one report, despite immediate withdrawal from a new treatment and institution of conventional combination chemotherapy, some patients had a poorer response rate and shorter survival than generally expected (11). Nevertheless, in general, inactive new agents have not subsequently impaired the results of standard salvage treatment.

Although evaluating new agents with preclinical activity in extensive stage untreated SCLC patients can more clearly identify activity, other investigators, particularly in Europe, have investigated new agents in previously treated patients. The approach is to test the new drug in particular groups of relapsed SCLC, e.g., those with a reasonable performance status without symptoms requiring a rapid tumor response. In the Lung Cancer Cooperative Group of the EORTC, it became clear that patients who had received relatively short-duration chemotherapy could still respond (50%) to rechallenge with identical chemotherapy if the recurrence had occurred at least 3 months after the end of the previous treatment and providing the patient had had a reasonable response to the initial chemotherapy. Patients who had been off chemotherapy for more than 2.6 months responded more frequently, as did patients who had been diagnosed more than 9 months before the beginning of new drug treatment. Discriminate analysis indicated that the time from prior chemotherapy was the most important factor (12). These data have been used to identify a group of previously treated patients who still had the possibility of responding to new active agents (12–14). Another approach to maximize the opportunity of identifying activity in previously treated patients is to lower the target response rate to 10% (10). Such an approach could result in more patients being treated in phase II studies with the possibility that more patients would be treated with an inactive drug. The threshold response rate of 20% can be maintained as an indicator of effectiveness if at least 40 patients who had previously responded to chemotherapy and who had a treatment-free interval of 3 months or more were enrolled (14). Therefore, in Europe Phase II new-agent studies in SCLC have usually been conducted in previously treated patients selected on the basis of the above criteria. Consideration of the patient population tested in new-drug evaluation is extremely important, so the response rate is placed in perspective and new drugs with activity are identified for subsequent more exhaustive evaluation.

TAXANES

Taxanes represent novel chemotherapeutic agents with different mechanisms of action from existing standard drugs used in SCLC. Paclitaxel and the synthetic analog docetaxel are the first new microtubule agents developed since the vinca alkaloids and exert cytotoxic effects by a unique mechanism of action. Both agents promote incorporation of tubulin into microtubules, which are rendered resistant to depolymerization, contrasting with vinca alkaloids, which just inhibit microtubule assembly. Compared with paclitaxel, docetaxel is more water-soluble and more potent at promoting tubule polymerization with a corresponding lower MTD (15). Both taxanes have shown important activity in ovarian cancer and breast cancer patients, and several studies have demonstrated significant activity in advanced non-small-cell lung cancer (15). Surprisingly, relatively few data exist for small-cell lung cancer. Indeed, in the recent Proceedings of the American Society of Clinical Oncology (1996) there were only four Phase I/II studies of paclitaxel for patients with small-cell lung cancer compared with 24 abstracts investigating non-small-cell lung cancer and none for docetaxel in small-cell lung cancer.

Two studies from the United States pointed to the activity of paclitaxel. The ECOG Phase II study used 250 mg/m^2 paclitaxel as a 24-h infusion in patients with untreated extensive stage disease. Treatment was given every 3 weeks up to four doses because of limited drug supply (16). The patients went on to receive salvage chemotherapy, cisplatin, and etoposide during or after the planned four courses of paclitaxel depending on response. Of 36 patients entered onto the study, 32 were assessable and 11 patients (34%) had a partial response. Another three patients had >50% tumor shrinkage, but there was no 4-week follow-up measurement and therefore these patients did not fulfill the response criteria. The median survival was 43 weeks, and 1-year estimated survival was 37%. The study demonstrated that paclitaxel was an active anticancer agent against SCLC. The high level of Grade IV toxicity (56% leukopenia) was due to the paclitaxel dose given as a 24-h infusion. A similar study was performed by the North Central Cancer Treatment Group, again in patients with extensive-stage SCLC with the same regimen of paclitaxel together with G-CSF and an unrestricted number of paclitaxel cycles. Patients who had disease progression or who had stable disease after six courses were switched to a platinum/etoposide regimen. There was a two-step Phase II study design (10). Initially 15 patients were assessed; if two or more responses were observed, then an additional 25 patients were enrolled. If 11 or fewer responses occurred in the 40 patients, the agent was rejected, as a response rate of at least 20% was expected. Thirty-seven patients of 43 were evaluable for a response with 15 PRs (17). The two studies confirmed the activity of paclitaxel in SCLC.

Docetaxel has also shown a wide spectrum of activity in preclinical antitumor models both in vitro and in vivo, and in Phase I testing there have been some hints of antitumor activity in patients with SCLC (18). In the only study yet published in full, docetaxel was assessed by the Early Clinical Trials Group of the EORTC (18). The Phase II trial comprised patients who had previously been treated with evidence of progressive disease. Patients were also eligible despite previous radiotherapy, providing that it was to a site other than that used to assess response. Docetaxel was given as 1-h intravenous infusion at 100 mg/m² every 21 days. Of 34 patients entered into the study, 27 had received previous chemotherapy, and eight previous radiotherapy. Seven partial responses which met the full criteria were recorded, and a further two in which the response was not maintained for 4 weeks, giving a 25% response rate for the 28 evaluable patients who had completed at least two courses of docetaxel. The major toxicity was neutropenia Grade IV (65% of patients) based on the worst grade per patient taken from weekly blood counts. Anemia and thrombocytopenia were much less severe. Seventy-six percent of patients had skin problems, ranging from erythema to desquamation, together with lethargy. There was only one serious infection despite the neutropenia. The response rate duration was up to 12 months. Although toxicity occurred, this was not untoward, and docetaxel demonstrated clear activity in this group of previously treated SCLC patients (19).

The only other European taxane study was performed by Dutch investigators, again in heavily pretreated patients. Paclitaxel was given at 175 mg/m^2 every 3 weeks as a 3-h IV infusion with the possibility of dose escalation to 200 mg/m^2. Sixteen patients—13 extensive-stage disease, three limited-stage disease, median performance status of 2, and a median of two previous chemotherapy regimens (range of two to four) were enrolled. The median time off therapy was only 5 weeks, and patients entered the study with early relapse, i.e., < 3 months off chemotherapy. Despite the unfavorable characteristics there were 11 dose escalations (no reductions) for a total of 33 courses. There was leukopenia of Grade III/IV on 23% of courses and thrombocytopenia on 11% of courses. One patient died of neutropenic sepsis. The main nonhematological toxicity was myalgia Grade III in three patients. Partial response occurred in five patients of 14 evaluable (35.7%) with a median survival of 16 weeks, range 5 to 53. Paclitaxel had significant activity in this heavily pretreated, clinically resistant group of SCLC patients, and further investigation is clearly warranted (20).

Evaluation of the taxanes in combination with other drugs known to have activity in SCLC both for patients who have relapsed or progressed on standard treatment and in previously untreated selected patients, is obviously required. The optimal dose and schedule of paclitaxel needs to be defined although 1-h infusions with docetaxel are effective. A number of potential combinations include taxanes with etoposide, cisplatin, ifosfamide, and the newer drugs such as topotecan and gemcitabine. Placlitaxel has also been given as a 1-h infusion together with carboplatin and low-dose daily etoposide in previously untreated patients with SCLC. The regimen was active and well tolerated in outpatients (21). Another approach has been to give high-dose paclitaxel 250 mg/m^2 and escalating doses of carboplatin with G-CSF/peripheral blood stem cell rescue (22) over multiple cycles. Another Phase I study from an Australian group examined two schedules of paclitaxel and oral etoposide for patients with lung cancer. Paclitaxel was escalated from 100 mg/m^2 given either on day 1 or on day 5 as a 3-h infusion with etoposide 100 mg orally on days 1 to 5. When the paclitaxel was given on day 5, dose-limiting myelosuppression occurred at a lower dose (160 mg/m^2) than when given on day 1 (200 mg/m^2) with a greater frequency of febrile neutropenia (23). Since paclitaxel is a radiosensitizer, studies are also needed to evaluate the drug with concurrent radiation treatment in better prognosis small-cell lung cancer patients (24).

Given the Phase I/II activity data in patients with poor prognostic characteristics, Phase II evaluations of taxanes in combination with other active agents, and with radiotherapy in patients with better-prognosis disease are needed. The use of higher doses with hemopoietic growth factor support will need to be evaluated. Easier methods of providing peripheral blood stem cell support by avoiding leucapheresis and cryopreservation through the use of whole-blood autotransfusions should also be considered (25,26).

Finally, randomized comparisons will be required to determine whether treatment with taxanes is superior to more standard therapy already in use. The taxanes represent an important new class of anticancer drugs and deserve much more attention in small-cell lung cancer.

REFERENCES

1. Moller Jenson O, Esteve J, Moller H, Renard H. Cancer in the European Community and its member states. Eur J Cancer 1990; 26: 1167–1256.
2. La Vecchia C, Lucchini F, Negri E, et al. Trends of cancer mortality in Europe, 1955–1989. II. Respiratory tract, bone, connective and soft tissue sarcomas and skin. Eur J Cancer 1992; 28:514–599.
3. Cancer Research Campaign. Lung Cancer and Smoking—UK. Factsheet 1996; 11.1.
4. Cerny T, Blair V, Anderson H, et al. Pretreatment prognostic factors and scoring system in 407 small-cell lung cancer patients. Int J Cancer 1987; 39:146–149.
5. Rawson NSB, Peto J. An overview of prognostic factors in small cell lung cancer. Br J Cancer 1990; 61:597–604.
6. Souhami RL, Law K. Longevity in small cell lung cancer. Br J Cancer 1990; 61:584–589.

7. Thatcher N, Clark PI, Girling DJ, et al. Medical Research Council Working Party. Comparison of oral etoposide and standard intravenous chemotherapy for small cell lung cancer: a stopped multicenter randomised trial. Lancet 1996; 348:563–566.

8. Souhami RI, Spiro SG, Rudd RM, et al. Five-day oral etoposide treatment for advanced small cell lung cancer: a randomised comparison with intravenous chemotherapy. J Natl Cancer Inst 1997; 89:577–580.

9. Ettinger DS, Finkelstein DM, Abeloff MD, et al. Justification for evaluating new anticancer agents in selected untreated patients with extensive-stage small cell lung cancer: an Eastern Cooperative Oncology Group randomized study. J Natl Cancer Inst 1992; 84:1077–1084.

10. Grant SC, Gralla RJ, Kris MG, et al. Single-agent chemotherapy trials in small cell lung cancer, 1970–1990: the case for studies in previously treated patients. J Clin Oncol 1992; 10:484–498.

11. Cullen MH, Smith SR, Benfield GFA, Woodroffe CM. Testing new drugs in untreated small cell lung cancer may prejudice the results of standard treatment: a Phase II study of oral idarubicin in extensive disease. Cancer Treat Rep 1987; 71:1227–1230.

12. Giaccone G, Donadio M, Bonardi G, et al. Teniposide in the treatment of small-cell lung cancer: the influence of prior chemotherapy. J Clin Oncol 1988; 6:1264–1270.

13. Giaccone G, Ferrati P, Donadio M, et al. Reinduction chemotherapy in small cell lung cancer. Eur J Cancer Clin Oncol 1987; 23:1697–1699.

14. Giaccone G. Identification of new drugs in pretreated patients with small cell lung cancer. Eur J Cancer Clin Oncol 1989; 25:411–413.

15. Francis PA, Kris MG, Rigas JR, et al. Paclitaxel (Taxol) and docetaxel (Taxotere): active chemotherapeutic agents in lung cancer. Lung Cancer 1995; 12(suppl 1):163–172.

16. Ettinger DS, Finkelstein DM, Sarma RP, Johnson DH. Phase II study of paclitaxel in patients with extensive-disease small-cell lung cancer: an Eastern Cooperative Oncology Group Study. J Clin Oncol 1995; 13:1430–1435.

17. Kirschling RJ, Jung SH, Jett JR. A phase II trial of taxol and GCSF in previous untreated patients with extensive stage small cell lung cancer (SCLC). Proc Am Soc Clin Oncol 1994; 13:326. Abstract 1076.

18. Extra J-M, Rousseau F, Bruno R, et al. Phase I and pharmacokinetic study of Taxotere (RP 56976; NSC 628503) given as a short intravenous infusion. Cancer Res 1993; 53:1037–1042.

19. Smyth JF, Smith IE, Sessa C, et al. Activity of docetaxel (Taxotere) in small cell lung cancer. Eur J Cancer 1994; 30A:1058–1060.

20. Smit EF, Kloosterziel C, Groen HJM, Postumus PE. A phase II study of paclitaxel (P) in heavily pretreated patients with small cell lung cancer (SCLC). Proc Am Soc Clin Oncol 1996; 15:394. Abstract 1192.
21. Hainsworth JD, McKay CE, Miller PS, Greco FA. Treatment of small cell lung cancer (SCLC) with paclitaxel (one hour infusion), carboplatin and low dose daily etoposide. Proc Am Soc Clin Oncol 1995; 14:384. Abstract 1197.
22. Shea T, Graham M, Bernard S, et al. Multiple cycles of high dose paclitaxel plus escalating doses of carboplatin with G-CSF (Filigrastim) and peripheral blood stem cell (PBSC) support. Proc Am Soc Clin Oncol 1995; 14:478. Abstract 1555.
23. Boyer M, Olver I, Millward M, Zalcberg J, et al. Phase I study of two schedules of taxol (T) and oral etoposide (E) in patients (pts) with small cell (SCLC) or non-small cell (NSCLC) lung cancer. Proc Am Soc Clin Oncol 1996; 15:390. Abstract 1177.
24. Tishler RB, Schiff PB, Geard CR, Hall EJ. Taxol: a novel radiation sensitizer. Int J Radiat Oncol Biol Phys 1992; 22:613–617.
25. Pettengell R, Woll PJ, Thatcher N, et al. Multicyclic, dose-intensive chemotherapy supported by sequential reinfusion of hematopoietic progenitors in whole blood. J Clin Oncol 1995; 13:148–156.
26. Woll PH, Lee SM, Lomax L, et al. Randomised phase II study of standard versus dose-intensive ICE chemotherapy with reinfusion of haemopoietic progenitors in whole blood in small cell lung cancer (SCLC). Proc Am Soc Clin Oncol 15:333. Abstract 957.

7

Phase III Experience with Paclitaxel in Non-Small-Cell Lung Cancer

North American Experience

Philip Bonomi
Rush University Medical Center, Chicago, Illinois

KyungMann Kim and David H. Johnson
Vanderbilt University Medical Center, Nashville, Tennessee

INTRODUCTION

Disseminated or locally recurrent disease will occur in the majority of non-small-cell lung cancer (NSCLC) patients. The outcome for this group of patients is disappointingly predictable, with a median survival of 4 months and a 1-year survival of approximately 10% in untreated patients (1,2). Investigators within the Eastern Cooperative Oncology Group (ECOG) have conducted a series of chemotherapy trials in patients who have Stage IV non-small-cell lung cancer. The initial studies (3,4) evaluated combination chemotherapy regimens which had produced response rates ≥ 25% in Phase II trials. Unfortunately, the earlier response rates observed with the combination regimens were not confirmed in the larger Phase III trials; the median survival duration was approximately 6 months, and the 1-year survival rate was 19% (5). Subsequently, ECOG conducted a transitional study in which single agents were compared to combination regimens (6). Despite the fact that the single agents produced significantly lower response rates compared to the combination regimens, the single agent, carboplatin, was associated with slightly longer survival than were the combination regimens; the survival duration for the other single agent, iproplatin, was virtually identical to the survival observed with the combination regimens.

Based on these observations, ECOG investigators decided to turn their attention to drug discovery. A series of new compounds were tested, and a response rate of 21% was observed with taxoll given at a dose of 250 mg/m^2 every 3 weeks (7). Simultaneously, investigators at M.D. Anderson Cancer Center observed 24% response rate with Taxol given at a dose of 200 mg/m^2 (8). Both groups (7,8) of investigators observed 1-year survival rates of approximately 40%.

Encouraged by the relatively high response rates and the 1-year survival rates observed, ECOG designed a Phase III trial to test Taxol's effect on survival. Etoposide-cisplatin was chosen as the reference regimen because it had produced the highest 1-year survival rate (25%) in previous ECOG trials (5). Two levels of Taxol (135 mg/m^2, and 250 mg/m^2) were combined with cisplatin. The decision to test the combination of Taxol and cisplatin rather than single-agent Taxol was based on the observation that cisplatin-containing regimens had been shown to produce a modest improvement in survival compared to supported care alone (9–11), database analyses conducted by the Southwest Oncology Group revealed a survival advantage for regimens that contained cisplatin (12). The higher dose of Taxol (250 mg/m^2) is identical to the dose used in our single-agent Phase II trial (7), the lower dose of Taxol (135 mg/m^2) was included because this dose and schedule of Taxol and cisplatin had produced significant improvement in survival in ovarian cancer (13). The major objective of this trial was comparison of survival durations for the Taxol regimens versus the reference regimen. Other objectives included comparison of response rates, and toxicity.

MATERIALS AND METHODS

Entry into this trial occurred between August 1993 and December 1994. Patients were required to have histologically or cytologically confirmed NSCLC. Patients whose tumors contained elements of small-cell carcinoma were excluded. Bidimensional measurable or evaluable disease was required. Other eligibility criteria included: ECOG performance status ≤ 1, no previous history of malignant disease with the exception of skin cancer or in situ carcinoma of the cervix, no Stage IIIb or Stage IV disease, and no brain metastases. In addition, patients were required to have adequate organ function, defined as follows: leukocyte count ≥ 4000/mm^3, platelets ≥ 100,000/mm^3; bilirubin ≤ 1.5 mg/dL, and serum creatinine ≤ 1.5 mg/dL. Patients with active infections were excluded, and patients who had received previous chemotherapy were not eligible. Patients were allowed to have previous radiation provided it had been completed ≥ 2 weeks prior to entry into this trial, and provided they had recovered from the side effects of radiation therapy. In addition, patients were not eligible if the only measurable lesion was within a previously radiated field. Other exclusion criteria included uncontrolled diabetes mellitus which was defined as a blood sugar > 200 mg/dL, uncontrolled hypertension, unstable angina, congestive heart failure, myocardial infarction within the previous year, and evidence of neuropathy by history of physical examination. Each patient gave written informed consent prior to entry into this study.

Treatment regimens were as follows: etoposide-cisplatin cisplatin 75 mg/m^2 IV over 1 h on day 1 plus etoposide 100 mg/m^2 IV over 45 min on days 1, 2, and 3; Taxol-cisplatin granulocyte colony-stimulating factor (G-CSF) cisplatin 75 mg/m^2 IV over 1 h on day 2 preceded by Taxol 250 mg/m^2 IV intravenously as a 24-h infusion on day 1, plus G-CSF 5 μg/kg subcutaneously beginning on day 3 and continuing until the granulocyte count was 10,000/mm^3; Taxol-cisplatin cisplatin 75 mg/m^2 IV over 1 h on day 2 preceded by Taxol 135 mg/m^2 given intravenously as a 24-h infusion starting on day 1. Each of the regimens was repeated every 21 days provided toxicity was acceptable and there was no evidence of disease progression. Patients were stratified according to the following parameters: (1) weight loss during the previous 6 months < 5% versus ≥ 5%; Stage IIIb versus Stage IV disease; bidimensional measurable disease versus evaluable disease.

History and physical examination and tumor measurements were performed before each treatment cycle as well as complete blood count and serum chemistries. Grades of toxicity and tumor responses were defined according to ECOG criteria (14). Fisher's exact test (15) was used in comparing response rates, and the Kruskal-Wallis (15) method was used in comparing degrees of toxicity. Survival estimates were calculated by the Kaplan-Meier (16) method, and log-rank (17) and Wilcoxon (17) methods were used for survival comparisons.

The study accrual goal was based on the following statistical considerations: first, we expected the Taxol containing regimens to be associated with longer survival than etoposide-cisplatin and therefore etoposide-cisplatin was compared to high-dose Taxol-cisplatin and G-CSF and to the lower-dose Taxol-cisplatin regimen using a two-sided $\alpha = 0.125$ test. With respect to comparison of the Taxol-containing regimens, we did not have an hypothesis about which regimen would be better and therefore a two-sided $\alpha = 0.025$ level was used in these analyses. The initial accrual goal was 480 patients. However, accrual occurred more rapidly than we had anticipated, and therefore the accrual goal was increased to 600 patients in order to improve the power to detect a survival difference between the regimens.

RESULTS

Between August 1993 and December 1994, 571 eligible patients were entered on this trial—194 on etoposide-cisplatin, 190 on Taxol-cisplatin-G-CSF, and 187 on Taxol-cisplatin. Patient characteristics are summarized in Table 1. The median age was 61.7 years, slightly more than one-third of the patients were women, and approximately 13% of the patients were non-Caucasian. In addition, one-third of the patients were completely asymptomatic, and approximately 75% of the patients had not lost more than 5% of their usual body weight during the 6 months before entry into the study. Stage IV disease was identified in 81% of the patients; the remaining 19% had Stage IIIb disease. The majority of the patients (78.6%) had measurable disease as opposed to evaluable disease.

There were no significant differences between the treatment arms with respect to the baseline patient characteristics.

Table 1 Patient Characteristics

Parameter	EC	TCG	TC
Median age (years)	61.7	60.5	62.5
% Males/females	65/35	63/37	62/38
% Caucasian/non-Caucasian	89/11	88/12	86/14
% PS 0/1	32/68	34/66	33/67
% Wt. loss $</\geq 5\%$	74/26	72/28	75/25
% IIIb/IV	19/81	19/81	19/81
% Meas/eval	79/21	78/22	79/21

Abbreviations: EC = etoposide-cisplatin; TCG = Taxol-cisplatin-G-CSF; TC = Taxol-cisplatin.

Response data are summarized in Table 2. The objective response rate (complete plus partial remissions) for etoposide-cisplatin was 12.4%, Taxol-cisplatin and G-CSF was 31.1%, and Taxol-cisplatin was 26.2%. The nominal p value for the observed difference response rates according to the Fisher's exact test was < 0.001 for etoposide-cisplatin versus Taxol-cisplatin-G-CSF, and for etoposide-cisplatin versus Taxol-cisplatin. The p value for the difference between Taxol-cisplatin-G-CSF versus Taxol-cisplatin was 0.308. Median response durations for each treatment was as follows: Etoposide-cisplatin 5.98 months, Taxol-cisplatin-G-CSF 6.47 months, and Taxol-cisplatin 5.52 months. Nominal p values for the observed differences in median response duration according to the log-rank

Table 2 Response Rates

Response	EC	TCG	TC	p value[a]
% CR	1	2.1	2.8	.001 EC v. TCG
% PR	11.3	28.9	23.5	.001 EC v. TC
% CR+PR	12.3	31.0	26.3	.308 TC v. TCG

Abbreviations: EC = etoposide-cisplatin; TCG = Taxol-cisplatin-granulocyte colony-stimulating factor; TC = Taxol-cisplatin.
[a]Fisher's exact test was used to compare the differences in response rates.

Table 3 Survival Results

Regimen	Median survival (months)	% 1-Year
EC	7.4	31.3
TCG	10.1	40.4
TC	9.6	37.3

Abbreviations: EC = etoposide-cisplatin; TCG = Taxol-cisplatin-granulocyte colony-stimulating factor; TC = Taxol-cisplatin.

test was 0.882 for etoposide-cisplatin versus Taxol-cisplatin-G-CSF, 0.64 etoposide-cisplatin versus Taxol-cisplatin, and 0.211 for Taxol-cisplatin-G-CSF versus Taxol-cisplatin.

Kaplan–Meier survival estimates were calculated after a median follow-up of 17.9 months, and a minimum potential follow-up of 16 months for all eligible patients. Median survival durations and 1-year survival rate are shown in Table 3. Kaplan-Meier survival estimates are depicted in Figures 1 to 3. Comparing the survival results for etoposide-cisplatin versus Taxol-cisplatin and G-CSF shows that the p values for log-rank in Wilcoxon analyses are 0.063 and 0.016, respectively (Fig. 1). The p values for log-rank and Wilcoxon comparisons for etoposide-cisplatin versus Taxol-cisplatin are 0.083 and 0.063, respectively (Fig. 2).

Comparison of the survival durations for Taxol-cisplatin-G-CSF versus Taxol-cisplatin reveals no significant differences (Fig. 3).

Hematological toxicity data are summarized in Table 4, and nonhematological toxicity data are depicted in Table 5. Comparisons of the various types of toxicity for each regimen are summarized in Table 6. The major toxicity was granulocytopenia with grade 4 toxicity occurring in the majority of patients. The incidence of proven infections and of temperature elevations ≥ 101°F were 7% to 9%. The observed differences in the degrees of toxicity using the Kruskal-Wallis test revealed a significantly higher percentage of grade 4 granulocytopenia in patients receiving lower-dose Taxol-cisplatin without G-CSF compared to etoposide-cisplatin and Taxol-cisplatin-G-CSF

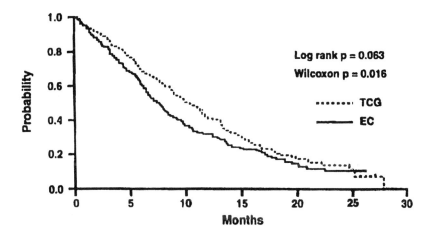

Figure 1   Kaplan-Meier plot for survival.

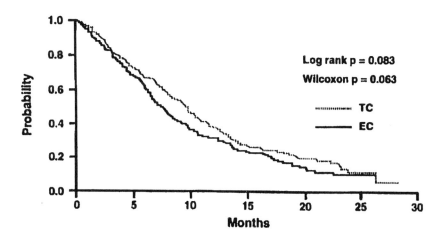

Figure 2   Kaplan-Meier plot for survival.

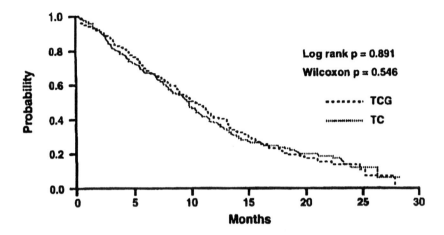

Figure 3   Kaplan-Meier plot for survival.

(Table 6). There were no significant differences in the rates of infection or febrile episode during granulocytopenia.

Grade 3 neurological toxicity, which was manifested predominantly as sensory abnormalities, occurred in 19% to 37% of the patients and was significantly more common on the Taxol-cisplatin-G-CSF arm. Severe nausea and vomiting was relatively infrequent.

Table 4   Hematological Toxicity

Parameter	EC	TCG	TC
% Grade 4 leukopenia	16	27	14
% Grade 4 granulocytopenia	55	65	74
% ≥ Grade 3 infection	8.5	9	7.4
% Grade 5 infection	1	3	1.5
% Grade 4 thrombocytopenia	5	5	.5
% ≥ Grade 3 anemia	27	20	20

Abbreviations: EC = etoposide-cisplatin; TCG = Taxol-cisplatin-granulocyte colony-stimulating factor; TC = Taxol-cisplatin.

Table 5 Nonhematological Toxicity

Parameter	EC	TCG	TC
% Grade 3 neurological	19	37	20
% Grade 4 N & V	6	8	9
% ≥ Grade 3 myalgias	0	7	.5
% Grade 5 cardiac[a]	0	.5	2.5
% Grade 5 all types	1	5	4.5

Abbreviations: EC = etoposide-cisplatin; TCG = Taxol-cisplatin-granulocyte colony-stimulating factor; TC = Taxol-cisplatin.
[a]Possibly treatment-related.

Grade 3 myalgia was significantly more common on the Taxol-cisplatin-G-CSF regimen. Possibly treatment-related cardiac toxicity was observed in 0.5% of patients on Taxol-cisplatin-G-CSF and in 2.5% of patients on Taxol-cisplatin. There were no significant differences in the possibly of treatment-related fatal cardiac events based on Fisher's test analyses in which grades 0 to 3 were compared to grades 4 and 5 toxicity.

DISCUSSION

Although Phase III trials in which best supportive care was compared to combination chemotherapy have shown conflicting results, based

Table 6 Toxicity Comparisons, Kruskal-Wallis Test p Values

Toxicity	EC vs. TCG	EC vs. TC	TC vs. TCG
Granulocytopenia	.08	<.001	.047
Infection	.50	.57	.25
Neurological	.002	.64	.005
Myalgias	<.001	<.001	<.001
Cardiac[a]	.68	.10	.38

Abbreviations: EC = etoposide-cisplatin; TCG = Taxol-cisplatin-granulocyte colony-stimulating factor; TC = Taxol-cisplatin.
[a]Fisher's exact test grades 0–3 vs. 4–5.

on a recent meta-analysis (1,2) it appears that chemotherapy produces a modest improvement in survival. In one of the meta-analyses improvement in survival was limited to the first 6 months (1); on the other study there was a slight improvement in the 1-year survival rate (2). Although database analyses conducted by the Southwest Oncology Group showed that treatment with cisplatin-containing regimens was associated with a slightly longer survival (12), the meta-analyses failed to identify a specific regimen which produced superior results (2). Similarly, until recently (18,19), trials in which single agents were compared to combination (6,20,21) regimens have failed to show a survival advantage for the combination regimens (6). In fact, as discussed earlier, in one of the trials (6), single-agent carboplatin was associated with slightly longer survival than three combination regimens.

Based on the large amount of data showing only minimal improvement in survival with combination chemotherapy (1,2), many investigators directed their efforts to drug discovery which has resulted in the identification of new agents with response rates > 20%—Vinorelbine, Taxol, Taxotere, Gemcitabine, Irinotecan, Topotecan, and Epirubicin (22).

With the availability of a relatively large number of new agents, investigators have initiated a number of Phase II trials testing combination regimens containing the new agents. In addition, several Phase III trials evaluating the effect of the new agents on survival have been conducted.

Vinorelbine has been studied most extensively. Three Phase III trials in which Vinorelbine-cisplatin was compared to either Vinorelbine (23) alone or cisplatin (19) alone have shown significantly higher response rates for the two-drug combinations, and two of these trials have shown improved survival for the two-drug combination, while in the third study no significant difference in survival was observed (24). Although one of the trials (23) failed to detect a survival advantage for the two-drug combination, the fact that in two of the trials (18,19) superior survival was observed for Vinorelbine-cisplatin versus either single agent alone is considerably different from earlier trials (20,21) in which survival durations for single agents and for combination regimens were not significantly different. In addition, in one of the studies Vinorelbine-cisplatin (18) was associated with significantly longer survival than another combination regimen (Vindesine-cisplatin).

Taxol is the other new agent which has been tested in Phase III trials. In our trial we observed significantly higher response rates and also longer survival which was marginally statistically significant for both Taxol regimens compared to etoposide-cisplatin. This is the first time that the Eastern Cooperative Oncology Group has observed a significant survival advantage for a combination regimen compared to other combination regimens.

A similar randomized trial was conducted by European investigators who compared Taxol-cisplatin was compared to cisplatin-Teniposide. This trial has also shown significantly higher response rates for Taxol-cisplatin (24). However, preliminary survival analyses have failed to show a difference between the regimens. The reason for this inconsistency in the survival results in the two randomized trials which evaluated Taxol-cisplatin is not readily apparent. However, ongoing Phase III trials evaluating Taxol-platinum combinations will provide additional data which could be evaluated in a meta-analysis.

Encouraged by the significantly higher response rates and the improved survival observed with both Taxol regimens, Eastern Cooperative Oncology Group investigators have initiated a Phase II trial which will evaluate combination regimens containing new agents. In this study Taxol (135 mg/m^2)-cisplatin will serve as the reference regimen which will be compared to Taxotere-cisplatin versus Taxol-carboplatin, versus Gemcitabine-cisplatin. Simultaneously, Vinorelbine-cisplatin, the other new regimen that has been associated with improved survival (18,19), is being compared to Taxol-carboplatin in Phase III trial being conducted by SWOG; Acute Leukemia Group B investigators are conducting a Phase III trial comparing Taxol alone to Taxol-carboplatin. While conducting the Phase III trials in Stage IV patients is important, we should also increase our efforts to study Taxol platinum combinations in combined modality treatments for Stage III patients.

REFERENCES

1. Grilli R, Oxman AD, Julian JA. Chemotherapy for advanced non-small-cell lung cancer: How much benefit is enough. J Clin Oncol 1993; 11:866.
2. Non-Small Cell Lung Cancer Collaborative Group. Chemotherapy in non-small cell lung cancer. A meta-analysis using updated data on individual patients from 52 randomized clinical trials. Br Med J 1995; 311:899–909.
3. Ruckdeschel JC, Finkelstein DM, Ettinger D, et al. Chemotherapy for metastatic non-small cell bronchogenic carcinoma: EST:2575, generation V-a randomized comparison of four cisplatin-containing regimens. J Clin Oncol 1985; 3:72.
4. Ruckdeschel JC, Finkelstein DN, Ettinger D, et al. A randomized trial of the four most active regimens for metastatic non-small-cell lung cancer. J Clin Oncol 1986; 4:14.
5. Finkelstein DM, Ettinger DS, Ruckdeschel JC. Long-term survivors in metastatic non-small cell lung cancer: an Eastern Cooperative Group study. J Clin Oncol 1986; 4:702.
6. Bonomi P, Finkelstein DN, Ruckdeschel JC, et al. Combination chemotherapy versus single agents followed by combination chemotherapy in stage IV non-small cell lung cancer: a study of the Eastern Cooperative Oncology Group. J Clin Oncol 1989; 7:1692.
7. Chang AT, Kim L, Glick J, et al. Phase II study of taxol, merbarone, and piroxantrone in stage IV non-small cell lung cancer. The Eastern Cooperative Oncology Group results. J Natl Cancer Inst 1993; 85:388.
8. Murphy WL, Fossella FV, Wenn RJ, et al. Phase II study of Taxol in patients with untreated advanced non-small cell lung cancer. J Natl Cancer Inst 1993; 85:384–387.
9. Rapp E, Pater JL, William A, et al. Chemotherapy can prolong survival in patients with advanced non-small-cell lung cancer: report of a Canadian multicenter randomized trial. J Clin Oncol 1988; 8:633.
10. Cellerino R, Tummorello D, Guidi F, et al. A randomized trial of alternating chemotherapy versus best supportive care in advanced non-small-cell lung cancer. J Clin Oncol 1991; 9:1453.
11. Cartei G, Cartei F, Cantene A, et al. Cisplatin-cyclophosphamide-mitomycin combination chemotherapy with supportive care versus supportive care alone for treatment of metastatic non-small-cell lung cancer. J Natl Cancer Inst 1993; 85:794.

12. Aslbain KS, Crowley JJ, LeBlanc MN, et al. Survival determinants in extensive non-small cell lung cancer. The Southwest Oncology Group experience. J Clin Oncol 1991; 9:1618.
13. McGuire WP, Hoskins WJ, Brady MF, et al. Cyclophosphamide and cisplatin compared with paclitaxel and cisplatin in patients with stage III and stage IV ovarian cancer. N Engl J Med 1996; 334:1–6.
14. Oken MM, Creech RH, Tormey DC, et al. Toxicity and response criteria of the Eastern Cooperative Oncology Group. Am J Clin Oncol 1982; 5:649–655.
15. Hays WI. Some Other Methods in Statistics. 3rd ed. New York: Holt Rinehart and Winston, 1981.
16. Kaplan FL, Meier P. Non-parametric estimation from incomplete estimation. J Am Stat Assoc 1958; 53:457–481.
17. Lagakos SW. Inference in survival analysis: non-parametric tests to compare survival distributions in statistics. In: Medical Researchers Editions. Miek V, Stanley KE, eds. New York: John Wiley and Sons, 1982.
18. LeChevalier T, Brisgand D, Doulliard JY, et al. Randomized study of vinorelbine and cisplatin versus vindesine and cisplatin versus vinorelbine alone in advanced non-small cell lung cancer: results of a European multicenter trial including 612 patients. J Clin Oncol 1994; 12:360.
19. Wozniak AJ, Crowley JJ, Balcerzak SP, et al. Randomized phase III trial of cisplatin versus cisplatin plus Navelbine in treatment of advanced non-small cell lung cancer: report of a Southwest Oncology Group Study (SWOG 9308). Proc Am Soc Clin Oncol 1996; 15:74.
20. Rosso R, Salvati F, Ardizzoni A, et al. Etoposide versus etoposide plus high-dose cisplatin in the management of advanced non-small cell lung cancer. Cancer 1990; 66:130.
21. Kawahara M, Furuse K, Nagohesa K, et al. A randomized study of cisplatin versus cisplatin plus vindesine for non-small-cell lung cancer. Cancer 1991; 68:74.
22. Lilenbaum RC, Green MP. Novel chemotherapeutic agents in the treatment of non-small-cell lung cancer. J Clin Oncol 1993; 11:1391.
23. DePierre A, Chastong CL, Quoix E, et al. Vinorelbine versus vinorelbine plus cisplatin in advanced non-small cell lung cancer. Ann Oncol 1994; 5:37–42.
24. Giaccone G, Splinter T, Postmus P, et al. Paclitaxel-cisplatin versus teniparide-cisplatin in advanced non-small-cell lung cancer. Proc Am Soc Clin Oncol 1996; 15:373.

8

Phase III Experience with Paclitaxel in Non-Small-Cell Lung Cancer

European Experience

Klaus Havemann and Martin Wolf
Zentrum fur Innere Medizin, Marburg-Lahn, Germany

INTRODUCTION

In recent years a large number of new cytotoxic agents with similar or unique mechanisms of action have been evaluated in patients with non-small-cell lung cancer. These agents, which include paclitaxel, docetaxel, the camptothecins, vinorelbine, and gemcitabine, have reported response rates of 20% to 40% with improvements in quality of life and symptoms related to the primary tumor. Especially paclitaxel has been extensively studied in recent years as single-agent or combination chemotherapy in NSCLC. Most of these studies have been performed in patients with inoperable locally advanced or metastatic disease (Stage IIIb and IV according to the UICC staging system). As single-agent chemotherapy the compound is able to achieve response rates of up to 30% and 1-year survival rates of about 40% (1,2). Using combination protocols with carboplatin or cisplatin, the response rates seem to be higher, reaching 40% to 60% of all patients, but its influence on survival is still questionable (3,4). In addition to the sole chemotherapy approach, in several studies the combination of paclitaxel treatment and radiotherapy has been investigated in patients with locally advanced inoperable disease. Paclitaxel arrests tumor cells in the M/G2 phase of the cell cycle, which represents the most radiation-sensitive cell cycle phase. Response rates of 50% to 75% have been reported (5,6), but the achievement of a complete remission still seems to be a rare event.

Despite the well-established activity of paclitaxel in the treatment of non-small-cell lung cancer, currently no mature data are evaluable on adjuvant or neoadjuvant treatment protocols in patients with potentially curable disease.

Although the results of the available Phase I and II trials in advanced non-small-cell lung cancer underline the high activity of paclitaxel in the treatment of this disease, its definitive value with respect to prolongation of survival is still an open question. To address this important issue only randomized trials comparing paclitaxel-containing regimens with non-paclitaxel-containing protocols (called standard treatment regimens) are necessary. To date only a very few of these randomized comparisons are evaluable, and the following section will summarize the experience in randomized trials in Europe which at the present time have only been published by the EORTC lung cancer study group.

THE EORTC EXPERIENCE

In July 1993 the EORTC started a randomized Phase II trial comparing the two drug combinations cisplatin/teniposide with cisplatin/paclitaxel in patients with advanced non-small-cell lung cancer. The main endpoints of this phase II trial were toxicity and response rates.

During the recruitment period from July 1993 to November 1994, 97 patients were included. The treatment protocol consisted either of cisplatin 80 mg/m^2 on day 1 plus teniposide 100 mg/m^2 days 1-3-5 or cisplatin 80 mg/m^2 on day 1 plus paclitaxel 175 mg/m^2 as a 3-h infusion prior to the cisplatin application. In both treatment arms six cycles were planned given in 3-week intervals. Table 1 summarizes the treatment plan.

The prognostic factors between the two treatment arms were well balanced. In a published interim analysis (7), 59 patients were evaluable. The median age was 57 years, 61% of the patients were

Table 1 Treatment plan of the EORTC Trial

Arm A:	Cisplatin	80 mg/m^2	day 1
	teniposide	100 mg/m^2	days 1, 3, 5
Arm B:	Cisplatin	80 mg/m^2	day 1
	paclitaxel	175 mg/m^2	day 1

Six cycles were given in 3-week intervals

male, and 83% had an ECOG performance status of 0 or 1. All patients had inoperable disease; 43% Stage IIIB and 57% Stage IV. The distribution of histology was 17% squamous carcinoma, 62% adenocarcinoma, and 21% large-cell carcinoma.

The hematological toxicity was much more pronounced in the teniposide-containing treatment arm. Leukopenia WHO Grade III to IV was seen in 60% vs. 17% of patients and thrombocytopenia Grade III to IV in 32% vs. 3%, respectively. Episodes of febrile neutropenia were reported in 25% of the patients receiving the teniposide-containing regimen, whereas this infection complications were not observed in the paclitaxel treatment group. On the other hand, myalgia Grade II to III was reported in 14% of the patients receiving paclitaxel whereas this side effect was not observed in the other treatment arm. There were no substantial differences in the incidences of peripheral neurotoxicity Grade II to III (15% vs. 20%), allergic reactions (4% vs. 7%), severe vomiting (16%), renal toxicity (3%), and alopecia (76%). Two treatment-related fatalities were observed—one in treatment arm A due to a septic shock, and one in treatment arm B due to pulmonary hemorrhage. The responses were extramurally reviewed and major tumor reduction was observed in three of 28 patients in the teniposide-containing and seven of 31 patients in the paclitaxel-containing treatment arm. Among the seven responses in treatment arm B, one complete remission was observed.

From these results it was concluded that the standard treatment arm produced similar activity and toxicity to what has been known from former clinical studies and that the new experimental arm was both tolerable and active. Based on these results of the randomized Phase II study, the EORTC then decided to move on into a randomized Phase III trial for which the major endpoint was comparison of survival between the two treatment arms. Additional endpoints of the Phase III trial were toxicity, response rates, and progression-free survival. Prolonging the recruitment period until February 1996, a total of 332 patients (166 in each arm) were randomized. As in the preceding Phase II trial the main prognostic parameters were well balanced between the two groups. The median age of the patients was 58 years, 17% were males, 19% of the patients had an ECOG performance status 0 to 1, and 62% had Stage IV disease. The distribution of the main prognostic factors between the two treatment groups is shown in Table 2.

The analysis of the toxicity shown in Table 3 (8) confirmed the former observations during the Phase II study period. The hematological toxicity was more severe and more common in the teniposide-containing regimen. Receiving this treatment 50% of the patients developed a grade III or IV leukopenia and almost 80% a grade III

Table 2 Distribution of the Main Prognostic Factors in the EORTC Trial (8)

	Cisplatin teniposide $n = 166\ (\%)$	Cisplatin paclitaxel $n = 166\ (\%)$
Males	71	70
Females	29	30
Performance status		
ECOG 0	34	33
1	57	55
2	9	12
Squamous cell	25	30
Adenocarcinoma	55	46
Large cell	20	24
Stage III	41	36
Stage IV	59	64

Table 3 Analysis of Toxicity in the EORTC Randomized Trial (8)

	Cisplatin teniposide	Cisplatin paclitaxel
Leukopenia WHO 3–4	69%	20%
Thrombocytopenia WHO 3–4	32%	2%
Febrile neutropenia	32%	1%
Neurotoxicity > WHO 1	16%	38%
Arthralgia/myalgia > WHO 1	3%	18%

or IV neutropenia. Also the incidence of severe thrombocytopenia was high and reached the 40% mark. This severe myelosuppression was responsible for treatment-related infections in a substantial number of patients (25%). On the other hand, the paclitaxel-containing treatment arm was associated with a relatively mild hematological toxicity consisting of an only 18% incidence of WHO grade III to IV leukopenia (54% WHO grade III to IV neutropenia) and an incidence of 3% WHO grade III to IV thrombocytopenia. Therefore, the frequencies for a treatment delays and dose reductions were substantially higher in the standard than in the new investigational treatment arm.

The nonhematological toxicity consisted of vomiting and alopecia in more than half of all patients with similar frequency in both arms. The incidences for peripheral neurotoxicity WHO grade > 1 were 38% vs. 16% and for arthralgia/myalgia WHO grade > 1 18% vs. 3% with higher incidences for the paclitaxel-containing treatment regimen. Low and similar frequencies of severe hypersensitivity reactions and cardiac toxicity were observed in both arms of the study. There have been five toxic deaths reported so far, two occurring in arm A and three in arm B.

To date 264 patients are evaluable; response rates were 47% in the paclitaxel-based treatment arm and 29% for those given cisplatin/teniposide. However, an extramural radiological response evaluation is still being carried out and therefore these response rates are still immature and may be expected to decrease slightly in both treatment arms. In the vast majority of the cases the responses were partial remissions. The median survival time of all patients is in the range of 9 months. It is still to early to draw conclusions about the comparison of the survival curves; however, so far the survival appears similar in the two treatment groups, but a longer follow-up is necessary to allow a conclusive comparison.

DISCUSSION

The European experiences with randomized Phase III trials testing paclitaxel-based chemotherapy protocols are still very restricted. Currently no other data from additional randomized trials are evaluable, so the randomized EORTC trial still represents the most important study in this therapeutic field. However, this study is still immature and needs a further follow-up to draw definitive conclusions, especially concerning the survival time of the patients. The first analysis of response rates confirm the experiences that have been seen in Phase II and Phase III trials in Europe and North America. Paclitaxel-cisplatin combination chemotherapy is an active treatment regimen for non-small-cell lung cancer, with response rates in the range of 40%. The toxicity of this treatment protocol in conventional doses is tolerable. The hematological toxicity usually is mild; dose-limiting side effects seem to be the occurrence of peripheral neurotoxicity and arthralgia/myalgia. The response rates of the paclitaxel-containing protocols are higher than the former so-called standard treatment regimens like PE or cisplatin-teniposide. This has been observed in the EORTC trial as well as in the large trial from the Eastern Cooperative Oncology Group comparing cisplatin/Taxol in two different dosages with the standard cisplatin-etoposide regimen (9). However, in both studies a definitive analysis of survival has not been performed. The interim analysis shows that there seems to be no substantial difference in survival in the EORTC trial, whereas the ECOG trial outlined a small survival benefit for the patients treated with the paclitaxel-based protocols.

    Therefore, today it is too early to decide whether the well-established chemotherapy regimens for treatment of non-small-cell lung cancer like cisplatin-etoposide may be replaced in future by a paclitaxel-containing therapy. Definitely there is a higher response rate with the new drug, but whether this higher response rate may be transferred to a prolongation of survival is still questionable. This discussion continues to take place, especially on the background of the high costs connected with the paclitaxel treatment. Even with this new and maybe most active single agent in the treatment of non-small-cell lung cancer, the achievement of a complete remission is a very rare event and very few if any patients will be cured by this treatment approach. This leads to the discussion as to whether the advanced stages of disease represent the appropriate patient populations for employing paclitaxel-based chemotherapy protocols. In our opinion this highly active compound should be used more intensively in patients with potentially curable disease, in either an adjuvant or neoadjuvant approach in patients with Stage II or Stage III A non-small-cell lung cancer.

REFERENCES

1. Chang AY, Kim K, Glick J, et al. A phase II study of Taxol, merbarone, and prioxantrone in stage IV non-small cell lung cancer: the Eastern Cooperative Oncology Group results. J Natl Cancer Inst 1993; 85: 388–394.
2. Murphy WK, Fossella FV, Winn RJ, et al. Phase II study of Taxol in patients with untreated advanced non-small cell lung cancer. J Natl Cancer Inst 1993; 85:384–387.
3. Langer CJ, Leighton JC, Comis RL, et al. Paclitaxel and carboplatin in combination in the treatment of advanced non-small cell lung cancer: a phase II toxicity, response, and survival analysis. J Clin Oncol 1995; 13: 1860–1870.
4. Muggia FM, Vafai D, Natale R, et al. Paclitaxel 3-hour infusion given alone and combined with carboplatin: preliminary results of dose-escalation trials. Semin Oncol 1995; 22(suppl 9):63–66.
5. Choy H, Safran H. Preliminary analysis of a phase II study of weekly paclitaxel and concurrent radiation therapy for locally advanced non-small cell lung cancer. Semin Oncol 1995; 22(suppl 9):55–57.
6. Wolf M, Faoro C, Görg C, et al. Paclitaxel and simultaneous radiation in the treatment of Stage IIIA/B non-small cell lung cancer. Semin Oncol 1996; 23(6)(suppl 16):108–112.

7. Giaccone G, Splinter TAW, Postmus P, et al. Teniposide-cisplatin vs. paclitaxel-cisplatin in advanced non-small cell lung cancer (NSCLC), results of a randomized phase II study of the EORTC-LCCG. Proc ASCO 1995; 14:1082.

8. Giaccone G, Splinter T, Postmus P, et al. Paclitaxel-cisplatin vs teniposide-cisplatin in advanced non-small cell lung cancer (NSCLC). Proc ASCO 1995; 15:1109.

9. Bonomi P, Kim K, Chang A, et al. Phase III trial comparing etoposide (E) cisplatin (C) versus Taxol (T) with cisplatin-G-CSF (G) versus Taxol-cisplatin in advanced non-small cell lung cancer. An Eastern Cooperative Oncology Group (ECOG) trial. Proc ASCO 1996; 15:1145.

9

Docetaxel Trials in Non-Small-Cell Carcinoma of the Lung

Richard J. Gralla
Ochsner Clinic, New Orleans, Louisiana

INTRODUCTION

Docetaxel, or Taxotere, is a new agent with established activity in several malignancies, including non-small-cell lung cancer. As with paclitaxel (Taxol), evidence of its single-agent activity is based on several single-arm Phase II trials rather than on random assignment comparison studies. Both taxoids share several preclinical and clinical features; however, differences exist that have the potential to result in varying clinical outcomes.

Both taxoids are derived from yew trees. Chemical synthesis from this source results in several active antitumor compounds including docetaxel and paclitaxel (1). Many in vitro and in vivo studies favored the antitumor and antimitotic activities of docetaxel over paclitaxel (2,3). Clinical development soon followed in Europe, Australia, Asia, and North America.

PHASE I TRIALS: DOSES AND TOXICITY

Docetaxel testing involved different schedules in typical escalating dosing steps. While the most prominent toxicity was myelosuppression, especially neutropenia, other side effects of a more unusual nature were observed in many of the trials. The majority of these side effects have been relatively easy to prevent or lessen.

The schedule felt to have the greatest clinical activity, based on dose intensity and on activity in preclinical models, was the every-3-week intravenous injection given over 1 h. The most common dose-limiting toxicity continued to be neutropenia at doses in the 75 mg/m^2 to 100 mg/m^2 range in the every-3-week trial schedule (4). In subsequent trials it became apparent that the most severe neutropenia occurred disproportionally in patients with chemically measurable hepatic dysfunction. Caution is now recommended for patients who have both elevated alkaline phosphatase (>2.5 times the upper limit of normal) and elevated transaminases (SGOT or SGPT at >1.5 times the upper limit of normal). Pharmacokinetic studies reinforced this recommendation with the finding of decreased clearance of docetaxel by 27% in patients with the above liver function abnormalities.

The most unexpected side effect was flud retention after several docetaxel administrations. This occurred, often as edema or pleural effusion, even in patients with evidence of major clinical response (5,6). The fluid retention was felt to be dose-limiting in some instances, although criteria for attenuating doses or stopping docetaxel were not established. Marked diminution of the fluid retention was found with the prophylactic use of corticosteroids. In one prospective evaluation, the problem was not symptomatic in any of the 33 patients receiving a twice-daily oral dose of 8 mg dexamethasone, beginning 1 day prior to docetaxel and continuing for 3 or 4 further days (7). Fluid accumulation or edema often cleared while patients continued on trial, with several of the patients receiving a year of every-3-week chemotherapy plus the dexamethasone regimen.

Other commonly reported side effects include cutaneous toxicity such as skin rash and nail changes. Investigators report that the former effect is markedly reduced with the corticosteroid regimen. Peripheral neuropathy is reported by appears to be less prominent than that occurring with paclitaxel, although formal comparison studies are lacking (4,5).

Hypersensitivity reactions, typically characterized by flushing or bronchospasm, occur occasionally within the first few minutes of starting a docetaxel infusion (4,5). Pretreatment is not required for this problem; hypotension is unusual, but has been reported. In most cases, after the hypersensitivity reaction the docetaxel infusion can be resumed without incident.

SINGLE-AGENT ACTIVITY IN NON-SMALL-CELL LUNG CANCER

Several Phase II studies have been completed in different settings using the every-3-week schedule of docetaxel. The results of six of these studies are outlined in Table 1. The consistent and high degree of activity is noteworthy (8–13), as is the median survival range of 7 to 13 months among the studies. It is also of interest that the response and survival rates were similar in two studies conducted at the same

Table 1   Single-Agent Activity of Docetaxel in Patients with Non-Small-Cell Lung Cancer Who Have Not Previously Received Chemotherapy

Chemotherapy	Patients entered	Major response rate[a]	Reference
Docetaxel 100 mg/m² every 3 weeks	29	28%	8
Docetaxel 75 mg/m² every 3 weeks	20	25%	9
Docetaxel 100 mg/m² every 3 weeks	41	32%	10
Docetaxel 100 mg/m² every 3 weeks	42	21%	11
Docetaxel 100 mg/m² every 3 weeks	48	27%	12
Docetaxel 60 mg/m² every 3 weeks	75	19%	13
Total	255	24%	(95% C.I. = 19% to 29%)

[a]Complete and partial response rates.

institution but using different doses of docetaxel (100 mg/m^2 or 75 mg/m^2) on the same schedule (8,9), and the survival rates were similar in a study using only 60 mg/m^2 of docetaxel (13). Although the studies are small, they suggest that the lower dose range may be equivalent while producing less toxicity. If this lower dose is equally effective, it could have relevance for combination trials.

Docetaxel has also been tested in patients who have previously been treated with cisplatin-containing regimens (12,14). The observed 17% response rate is remarkable in that no other single agent has been reported to produce a major response rate over 10% in previously treated patients in repeated trials. Even with combination chemotherapy, studies showing useful activity in this setting are rare. One study of 29 patients noted a 19% partial response rate with the combination of mitomycin plus vindesine in patients who had prior treatment with cisplatin (15). Of the newer single agents used in non-small-cell lung cancer, such as paclitaxel or vinorelbine, response rates in previously treated patients have generally been low, especially in the larger trials (16,17).

Table 2 lists the antitumor activity seen in the studies enlisting patients with prior cisplatin chemotherapy. The estimated median survival of 8 months is unusual in previously treated patients with advanced non-small-cell lung cancer. It must be noted that these patients had good prognostic factors at the time of enlistment,

Table 2 Major Response Rates[a] in Patients with Non-Small-Cell Lung Cancer Who Were Previously Treated with Cisplatin Regimens

Chemotherapy	Patients entered	Major response rate	Reference
Docetaxel 100 mg/m^2 every 3 weeks	44	21%	12
Docetaxel 100 mg/m^2 every 3 weeks	44	14%	14
Mitomycin + vindesine	29	17%	15

[a]Complete and partial response rates.

with the majority being women and with a high overall performance status (12,14). Nonetheless, such findings are unusual and deserve attention. Do these results indicate that future studies should report responses according to whether or not patients responded to their initial chemotherapy, as is now done in second-line studies in patients with small-cell lung cancer? Do the results suggest that docetaxel is not largely corss-resistant with cisplain, which would be important in the design of combination studies?

At present, random-assignment studies with docetaxel have not been completed. Two trials based on the data from the studies with previously treated patients are continuing to enlist patients. The first of these is an international study in which patients previously treated with cisplatin regimens are assigned to receive either docetaxel or supportive care. Enlistment in this study has been relatively slow, while the second trial in this population comparing docetaxel with either vinorelbine or ifosfamide, has understandably had more rapid case accession. These trials have been planned to enter a large number of patients; in addition to clarifying the role of docetaxel in a second-line setting, they will also outline the activity of the comparator agents in previously treated patients.

RATIONALE FOR COMBINATION STUDIES WITH DOCETAXEL

Several reasons are apparent for using this agent in combination chemotherapy; however, the choice of agents to use with docetaxel is more complicated. The docetaxel single-agent activity in non-small-cell lung cancer is encouraging. Activity with docetaxel after treatment with cisplatin implies a lack of cross resistance and makes this latter agent a particularly attractive candidate for study with docetaxel.

The results of recent studies and analyses have given further strength for using cisplatin in combination regimens. First, studies using the meta-analysis methodology have indicated that regimens containing cisplatin, as outlined in earlier trials (18–20), have a modest but significant impact on survival in patients with advanced lung cancer (21,22). Second, large multicenter random-assignment trials have shown that the agents added to cisplatin (when the dose of cisplatin is kept the same in comparison arms) can also influence survival (23–25).

The side-effects profile of cisplatin makes it both logical and difficult for use with docetaxel. Cisplatin is attractive for combining with any agent due to its relatively mild degree of myelosuppression. This factor often allows the cisplatin and the accompanying agents to be given at or near their full Phase II single-agent doses. Conversely, the risks of emesis, nephrotoxicity, and fatigue make cisplatin a difficult agent. Good supportive care techniques have reduced the former risks (26,27); however, the asthenia associated with this agent has not been easy to control.

For both laboratory and clinical reasons, several other agents could be useful in combination with docetaxel. With newer agents demonstrating activity in non-small-cell lung cancer, many regimens are possible. The vinca alkaloids are attractive based on their confirmed activity in this malignancy, the theoretical appeal of interfering with microtubule assembly by two mechanisms of action, and the laboratory observation of synergy when given within 24 h of docetaxel. For these reasons, dose-finding studies with docetaxel and vinorelbine are now being conducted.

Gemcitabine activity has been shown in both single-agent and combination trials in lung cancer. This agent has a favorable side-effects profile and is easily given on an outpatient basis, making it an interesting agent to use with docetaxel. Single-arm studies indicating activity of paclitaxel plus carboplatin have encouraged similar trials with the later agent added to docetaxel. The potential difficulty with carboplatin and with vinorelbine is that both produce more myelosuppression than the other agents in their respective classes. The increased myelosuppression, despite the use of growth factors, may make combinations with docetaxel more toxic than regimens using the congeners.

While combinations with several other agents in addition to docetaxel could be interesting, the greatest clinical experience has been with cisplatin. The results of these studies will be discussed in the next section.

DOCETAXEL PLUS CISPLATIN TRIALS

Three trials have now been reported that combine docetaxel with cisplatin in patients with advanced non-small-cell lung cancer who are previously untreated with chemotherapy. Several similarities exist among these trials, allowing for a better overall view of the activity of the regimen. These similarities include patient characteristics that are largely similar in all studies. All three studies share an every-3-week treatment regimen and at least one common dose level in each trial. Each study incorporated both Phase I and Phase II objectives. The trials were each single-institution studies, conducted in the United States, France, and Australia.

While generally similar, there were some differences among the trials that are worth noting. Some different combination dose levels were explored. The Australian trial continued with both the docetaxel and the cisplatin given every 3 weeks, while the French and the U.S. studies administered the docetaxel every 3 weeks but gave the cisplatin on days 1 and 22 and then every 6 weeks. The preliminary results of the trials, as well as some of the differences, are outlined in Table 3.

Table 3 Docetaxel + Cisplatin Combination Studies in Patients with No Prior Chemotherapy and Stage IIIB or IV Non-Small-Cell Lung Cancer

	France	Australia	U.S.
Docetaxel dose (mg/m^2)	75	75	65 to 85
Cisplatin dose (mg/m^2)	100	75	75 to 100
Number of patients	51	47	33
Major response rate[a]	30%	39%	52%
Median survival	10 months	10 months	10 months
Reference	29	30	28

[a]Major response = complete + partial.
Docetaxel given every 3 weeks in all trials.
Cisplatin given every 3 weeks in the Australian trial.
Cisplatin given days 1 and 22 and then every 6 weeks in the French and U.S. trials.

The U.S. trial explored four dose levels (28). The only dose-limiting toxicity was neutropenia. With the prophylactic dexamethasone regimen, outlined earlier in this report, fluid retention and rash were not of clinical significance in the 33 patients treated, with several receiving docetaxel for up to 1 year (8). In the Phase I portion, it was concluded that 85 mg/m^2 of docetaxel was too high when combined with cisplatin. When giving cisplatin at 100 mg/m^2, the investigators favor using docetaxel at 65 mg/m^2, although doses of 75 mg/m^2 of docetaxel can be given. If the latter dose of docetaxel is used, this trial recommends a cisplatin dose of 75 mg/m^2. The 50% complete and partial response rate observed (with the majority of patients treated at 75 mg/m^2 of each agent) was encouraging, as was the projected median survival of 10 months. All patients were treated on an outpatient basis; neither growth factors nor prophylactic antibiotics were used.

The French trial used the same dosing interval for both agents as in the U.S. study. Of interest, the French study found less neutropenia than any of the other studies and favored docetaxel at 75 mg/m^2 plus cisplatin 100 mg/m^2 (29). While the major response rate observed in this trial (30%) was the lowest among the three, it should be realized that this trial had the largest proportion of patients with Stage IV extent (85%); nonetheless, the median survival is similar to the other studies and is projected to be 10 months.

A response rate intermediate between the French and U.S. figures was reported in the Australian study, as was the amount of neutropenia (30). This group concluded that the 75 mg/m^2 dose of both agents with each given every 3 weeks was the Phase II level. Similar to the other studies, their preliminary analysis predicts a 10-month median survival.

DOCETAXEL COMBINED WITH OTHER AGENTS

As previously mentioned, many combinations with docetaxel—in addition to those with cisplatin—are of interest. There is an ongoing study adding vinorelbine to docetaxel. The initial plan used the every-3-week docetaxel schedule with vinorelbine given on days 1, 2, and 3.

This schedule did not permit favorable dose intensity, and the authors are now investigating an every-2-week schedule of both docetaxel and vinorelbine (31). In that both these agents have activity in breast cancer, including among women previously treated with anthracyclines, this regimen could have a wide range of interest. Combination regimens with the other vinca alkaloids could be of interest in a variety of tumors, including lymphomas. Vincristine could be a reasonable agent to test with docetaxel, given its low level of myelosuppression and the possibly lower degree of peripheral neutropathy observed with docetaxel compared with paclitaxel.

Another study has the design of adding carboplatin to docetaxel with the use of growth factors (32). This trial is continuing, but the investigators expect to establish the Phase II dose in the near future. This combination, as well as the docetaxel plus cisplatin regimen, would be expected to be active in ovarian carcinoma.

DISCUSSION

To date, no random-assignment trials with docetaxel combination regimens have been reported. This is appropriate in that data from the initial combination studies have only recently become available.

A question that can be raised with each of the taxoids concerns the recommended doses of the agents used singly. With paclitaxel there appears to be a broad range of doses suggested in single-agent and in combination trials. In at least one recent trial in non-small-cell lung cancer, higher doses of paclitaxel did not appear to have much impact on the therapeutic activity (33). Is the same true for docetaxel? The Phase II studies conducted consecutively at Memorial Hospital indicate similar survival rates for 75 mg/m^2 and for 100 mg/m^2 (9,10). If further studies confirm this observation, then lower docetaxel doses would be indicated. Lower doses of both taxoids would be safer and easier to use in combination regimens. It would also mean that using fully effective taxoid doses in combination regimens would be more easily achieved.

As discussed in the prior section of this paper, many interesting combinations with docetaxel are possible. In that docetaxel has a broad range of antitumor activity, these combinations could have relevance for a variety of malignancies.

Putting current taxoid combination regimens into a reasonable context is difficult at this time when few random-assignment studies have been completed. There are, however, a few considerations that should be kept in mind. First, many current trials enlist patients with better prognostic factors than was true in the 1980s. This point is illustrated by the recent ECOG trial comparing paclitaxel plus cisplatin combinations with etoposide plus cisplatin (33). Entry criteria for that study required a high performance status, and some patients had stage II extent. In general, patients on the docetaxel plus cisplatin Phase II studies were of good performance status, with many patients having Stage III extent (except in the French trial). These trials are contrasted to the *British Medical Journal* meta-analysis examining the chemotherapy trials comparing older cisplatin plus vinca alkaloid regimens in which approximately 80% of patients had distant metastases, and several studies admitted patients of lower performance status (21).

Second, it should be noted that the 7-month median survival for the slightly inferior etoposide plus cisplatin arm in the ECOG study (33) was nearly identical to the same regimen in the multicenter European trial (24), in which the older MVP regimen (mitomycin plus vindesine plus cisplatin) with a 10-month median survival performed as well as the best results reported with taxoid combinations in similar random-assignment trials (33).

It is encouraging to have a variety of new agents, including the taxoids, with activity in non-small-cell lung cancer. The interesting early results with docetaxel and with paclitaxel are thought-provoking. Do we know how to use these agents in the best possible ways? Do other combinations with these agents have the potential for enhanced activity and greater ease of use? Whether the currently obtained results are superior to those recently reported with the best of the older regimens (24), which can be composed completely of lower cost generically available agents (such as MVP with high-dose cisplatin), can only be answered by large, random-assignment trials.

REFERENCES

1. Mangatal L, Adeline MT, Guenard D, Gueritte-Voegelein F, Potier P. Application of the vicinal oxymination reaction with assymetric induction to the hemisynthesis of taxol and analogues. Tetrahedron 1989; 45:4177–4190.
2. Gueritte-Voegelein F, Guenard D, Lavelle F, et al. Relationships between the structure of Taxol analogues and their antimitotic activity. J Med Chem 1991; 34:992–998.
3. Ringel I, Horwitz SB. Studies with RP 56976 (Taxotere): a semisynthetic analogue of Taxol. J Natl Cancer Inst 1991; 83:288–291.
4. Burris H, Irvin R, Kuhn J, et al. Phase I clinical trial of Taxotere administered as either a 2-hour or 6-hour intravenous infusion 3 weeks. J Clin Oncol 1993; 11:950–958.
5. Tomiak E, Piccart MJ, Karger J, et al. Phase I study of docetaxel administered as a 1-hour intravenous infusion on a weekly basis. J Clin Oncol 1994; 12:1458–1467.
6. Francis P, Schneider J, Hann L, et al. Phase II trial of docetaxel in patients with platinum-refractory advanced ovarian cancer. J Clin Oncol 1994; 12:2301–2308.
7. Rittenberg CN, Gralla RJ, Cole JT, et al. Preventing docetaxel-induced fluid retention: the efficacy of corticosteroids. Proc Am Soc Clin Oncol 1996; 15:531.
8. Francis PA, Rigas JR, Kris MG, et al. Phase II trial of docetaxel in patients with stage III and IV non-small cell lung cancer. J Clin Oncol 1994; 12:1232–1237.
9. Miller VA, Rigas JR, Kris MG, et al. Phase II trial of docetaxel given at a dose of 75 mg/m^2 with prednisone premedication in non-small lung cancer. Proc Am Soc Clin Oncol 1994; 13:364.
10. Fossella FV, Lee JS, Murphy WK, et al. Phase II study of docetaxel for recurrent or metastatic non-small cell lung cancer. J Clin Oncol 1994; 12:1238–1244.
11. Cerny T, Kaplan S, Pavlidis N, et al. Docetaxel (Taxotere) is active in non-small cell lung cancer: a phase II trial of the EORTC early clinical trials group (ECTG). Br J Cancer 1994; 70:384–387.
12. Burris HA, Eckardt J, Fields S, et al. Phase II trials of Taxotere in patients with non-small cell lung cancer. Proc Am Soc Clin Oncol 1993; 12:335.
13. Kunitoh H, Koshiro W, Taisuke O, et al. Phase II trial of docetaxel in previously untreated advanced non-small cell lung cancer: a Japanese Cooperative Study. J Clin Oncol 1996; 14:1649–1655.

14. Fossella FV, Lee JS, Shin DM, et al. Phase II study of docetaxel (Taxotere) for advanced or metastatic platinum-refractory non-small cell lung cancer. J Clin Oncol 1995; 13:645–651.

15. Kris MG, Gralla RJ, Kelsen DP, et al. Trial of Vindesine plus Mitomycin in stage III non-small cell lung cancer. An active out-patient regimen. Chest 1985; 87:368–372.

16. Murphy WK, Fossella FV, Winn RJ, et al. Phase II study of Taxol in patients with untreated advanced non-small cell lung cancer. J Natl Cancer Inst 1993; 85:384–388.

17. Ruckdeschel J, Wagner H, Williams C, et al. Second-line chemotherapy for resistant, metastatic, non-small cell lung cancer (NSCLC): the role of Taxol (TAX). Proc Am Soc Clin Oncol 1994; 13:357.

18. Gralla RJ, Casper ES, Kelsen DP, et al. Cisplatin and Vindesine combination chemotherapy for advanced carcinoma of the lung: a randomized trial investigating two dosage schedules. Ann Intern Med 1981; 95:414–420.

19. Kris MG, Gralla RJ, Kalman LA, et al. Randomized trial comparing Vindesine plus cisplatin with Vinblastine plus cisplatin in patients with non-small cell lung cancer with an analysis of methods of response assessment. Cancer Treat Rep 1985; 69:387–395.

20. Rapp E, Pater J, William A, et al. Chemotherapy can prolong survival in patients with advanced non small cell lung cancer. Report of a Canadian multicenter randomized trial. J Clin Oncol 1988; 6:633–641.

21. Non-Small Cell Lung Cancer Collaborative Group. Chemotherapy in non-small cell lung cancer: a meta-analysis using updated data on individual patients from 52 randomised clinical trials. BMJ 1995; 311:899–909.

22. Souquet PJ, Chauvin F, Boissel JP, et al. Polychemotherapy in advanced non-small cell lung cancer: a meta-analysis. Lancet 1993; 342:19–21.

23. LeChevalier T, Brisgand D, Douillard JY, et al. Randomized study of Vinorelbine and cisplatin versus Vindesine and cisplatin versus Vinorelbine alone in advanced non-small cell lung cancer: results of a European multicenter trial including 612 patients. J Clin Oncol 1994; 12: 360–367.

24. Crino L, Clerici M, Figoli F, et al. Chemotherapy of advanced non-small cell lung cancer: a comparison of three active regimens. A randomized trial of the Italian Oncology Group for Clinical Research (G.O.I.R.C.). Ann Oncol 1995; 6:347–353.

25. Wozniak AJ, Crowley JJ, Balcerzak SP, et al. Randomized phase III trial of cisplatin (CDDP) vs. CDDP plus Navelbine (NVB) in treatment of advanced non-small cell lung cancer (NSCLC): report of a Southwest

Oncology Group STudy (SWOG-9308). Proc Am Soc Clin Oncol 1996; 15:374.

26. Gralla RJ. Adverse effects of treatment: antiemetic therapy. In: Devita VT, Hellman S, Rosenberg SA, eds. Cancer, Principles and Practices of Oncology. Vol. IV. Philadelphia: Lippincott, 1993:2338–2348.

27. Hayes DM, Cvitkovic E, Goldberg RB, et al. High-dose cisplatinum diaminedichloride: amelioration of renal toxicity by mannitol diuresis. Cancer 1977; 39:1372–1381.

28. Cole JT, Gralla RJ, Marques CB, et al. Phase I-II study of cisplatin + docetaxel (Taxotere) in non-small cell lung cancer (NSCLC). Proc Am Soc Clin Oncol 1995; 14:357.

29. ESMO, 1996.

30. Zalcberg JR, Bishop JF, Millward MJ, et al. Preliminary results of the first phase II trial of docetaxel in combination with cisplatin in patients with metastatic or locally advanced non-small cell lung cancer (NSCLC). Proc Am Soc Clin Oncol 1995; 14:351.

31. Kris MG, Miller VA, Grant SC, et al. Trials of docetaxel (Taxotere) in patients with advanced non-small cell lung cancer at Memorial Sloan-Kettering Cancer Center. 4th Central European Lung Cancer Conference, 1996.

32. P. Belani, personal communication.

33. Bonomi P, Kim K, Chang A, et al. Phase III trial comparing etoposide (E) cisplatin (C) versus Taxol (T) with cisplatin-G-CSF (G) versus Taxol-cisplatin in advanced non-small cell lung cancer. An Eastern Cooperative Oncology Group (ECOG) Trial. Proc Am Soc Clin Oncol 1996; 15:382.

10

Single-Agent Paclitaxel as Second-Line Chemotherapy for Resistant, Metastatic, Non-Small-Cell Lung Cancer

Linda L. Garland, John C. Ruckdeschel, Henry Wagner, Jr., Charles C. Williams, Jr., Gail Shaw, Scott J. Antonia, Mary Heise, Jane Hilstro, and Alan Cantor
H. Lee Moffitt Cancer Center and Research Institute, Tampa, Florida

INTRODUCTION

Combination chemotherapy utilizing a platinum compound combined with a topoisomerase II inhibitor or mitotic spindle poison has been the mainstay of treatment for metastatic NSCLC in patients with good performance status (1). Despite response rates in the range of 20% to 30%, these combinations have yielded only modest gains of 2 to 3 months in median survival and a 15% improvement in 1-year survival, compared to patients treated with best supportive care.

Disease that has progressed after platinum-based therapy is typically refractory to second-line chemotherapy. Second-line chemotherapy generally yields response rates of less than 15%; these responses are often short-lived and are achieved at the expense of significant toxicity.

Over the last decade, intense efforts in drug development have yielded several new classes of highly active cytotoxic agents, including the taxanes. Paclitaxel (Taxol; Bristol-Meyers Squibb Company, Princeton, NJ), a taxane derived from the Pacific yew *Taxus brevifolia* that acts uniquely to polymerize mitotic spindle microtubules, was shown in efficacy studies to be a highly active single agent in NSCLC. In chemo-naive patients with stage IV disease at diagnosis or metastatic disease following local therapy for early-stage disease, response rates of >20% and 1-year survivals of 30 to 40% have been achieved (2,3).

At the time paclitaxel first became commercially available, the standard of care for good performance status patients with stage IV NSCLC included treatment with etoposide-cisplatin (4,5), vinblastine-cisplatin, or variations of mitomycin-vinblastine-cisplatin (6,7). Patients who progressed on these regimens and remained in excellent performance status had few options. The encouraging efficacy and toxicity profile of paclitaxel led our group to use it as single-agent, second-line therapy for metastatic NSCLC that had progressed after platinum-based chemotherapy. We then performed a retrospective review in order to define the toxicity, response, and survival for this group of patients.

PATIENTS AND METHODS

Patients had histologically proven non-small-cell lung cancer including adenocarcinoma, squamous cell, large-cell, and bronchoalveolar cell types. All patients had metastatic disease and had received prior chemotherapy with at least one platinum-containing regimen; all had evidence of progressive disease that was bidimensionally measurable or assessable. Patients had an ECOG performance status of 0 to 2, an expected survival of ≥ 12 weeks, adequate bone marrow reserve (absolute granulocyte count ≥ 2000/mL, platelet count $\geq 100,000$/mL, hemoglobin ≥ 10 g/dL), and adequate renal and liver function (serum creatinine ≤ 1.5 mg/dL and bilirubin, alkaline phosphatase, and aspartate aminotransferase < 1.5 times normal). Patients with active cardiac disease (uncontrolled arrhythmias or congestive heart failure) were excluded from this treatment. Patients who had had prior chest radiotherapy or radiotherapy to other sites had measurable disease not within the radiation port. At least 4 weeks had elapsed between radiotherapy and treatment with paclitaxel.

Chemotherapy was administered on day 1 of a 28-day cycle with a 24-h infusion of paclitaxel 125 to 250 mg/m^2 depending on extent of prior chest radiotherapy and renal function. Premedication included dexamethasone 20 mg, diphenhydramine 50 mg, and cimetidine 300 mg intravenously 30 min prior to paclitaxel administration. Toxicities were evaluated prior to each cycle of chemotherapy according to the WHO common toxicity criteria. A 20% dose reduction was made for hematological toxicity including febrile neutropenia, grade 4 thrombocytopenia, and any grade 4 nonhematological toxicity encountered during the preceding cycle of chemotherapy. Granulocyte colony-stimulating factor use was flexible and at the discretion of the investigator. Assessment of response was based on Eastern Cooperative Oncology Group response criteria. Time to progression and survival were measured from the first day of treatment.

RESULTS

Between January and December 1993, 16 patients were treated as above. Patient characteristics are outlined in Table 1. The median age of patients was 62.5 years. All patients had stage IV NSCLC at presentation or had developed metastatic disease after therapy for early-stage disease. More than one-third of patients had an ECOG performance status of 2. All patients had been previously treated with a platinum compound (11 with cisplatin, four with carboplatin, one with both compounds). Seven of 16 patients (44%) had prior treatment with thoracic radiotherapy.

Thirty-seven cycles of paclitaxel were administered; six patients received one cycle; five received two cycles; and five patients received between three and six cycles. The starting paclitaxel dose was 250 mg/m^2 for 11 patients, 200 mg/m^2 for four patients, and 125 mg/m^2 for one patient with renal insufficiency and prior thoracic radiotherapy. Dose reductions for toxicity were required for five patients. Growth factor was administered in 6 of 16 patients.

Table 1 Patient Characteristics

Characteristic	No. of patients
Total	16
Median age (yr)	62.5
Range	36–75
Sex	
Male	9
Female	7
ECOG performance status	
0	1
1	8
2	7
Histology	
Adenocarcinoma	8
Squamous	3
Large cell	2
Bronchoalveolar	3
No. prior chemotherapies	
1	11
2	3
3	2
Prior radiotherapy	8
Thoracic radiotherapy	7

Abbreviation: ECOG, Eastern Cooperative Oncology Group.

Fifteen of 16 patients were evaluable for toxicity (one patient received a single cycle of drug and was lost to follow-up for evaluation for toxicity). One patient died 48 h after the first paclitaxel infusion, due to unclear causes. The major toxicity was myelosuppression (Table 2), with 10 patients (67%) experiencing grade 3 or 4 leukopenia. Anemia and thrombocytopenia were generally mild. Infection-related toxicities were rare, with one episode of febrile neutropenia and one pneumonia. There were no hypersensitivity reactions. One patient had mild infusion-related hypotension; no other cardiac toxicities were seen. There was little or no gastrointestinal toxicity, with four patients (26%) experiencing mild esophagitis. The

Table 2 Toxicity

	Patients (%)	
	Grade 3	Grade 4
Leukopenia	7 (47)	3 (20)
Anemia	1 (7)	0 (0)
Thrombocytopenia	1 (7)	0 (0)
Allergic	0 (0)	0 (0)
Cardiac	0 (0)	0 (0)
Nausea/emesis	1 (7)	0 (0)
Esophagitis	0 (0)	0 (0)
Hepatic	1 (7)	0 (0)
Neurological		
Paresthesias	0 (0)	0 (0)
Neurosensory	0 (0)	0 (0)
Neuropsychiatric	0 (0)	0 (0)
Motor weakness	0 (0)	0 (0)
Fatigue	4 (27)	2 (13)
Pulmonary	2 (13)	0 (0)
Infection	1 (7)	0 (0)
Musculoskeletal	7 (47)	1 (7)

second most significant toxicity was a delayed fatigue syndrome which was experienced by two-thirds of patients overall, and was profound in six patients (40%). Fatigue was the dose-limiting toxicity for two patients. Three patients experienced musculoskeletal toxicities including bone pain, myalgias, in one patient, severe muscle cramping that was dose-limiting. Neurotoxic effects were mild, with grade 1 paresthesias noted in about one-quarter of patients, and headache and depression in one patient each.

Response data are available for 14 of 16 registered patients (Table 3). Three patients (21%) had partial responses, one of which was long-lived (8.8 months). Two patients each had minor responses and prolonged stable disease. Seven patients (50%) had progressive disease, including one patient who had a partial response which lasted less than 2 months. Time to progression is shown for the study group

Table 3   Response to Treatment ($n = 14$)

	No. of patients (%)
Complete response	0 (0)
Partial response	3 (21)
Minor response	2 (14)
Stable disease	2 (14)
Progressive disease	7 (50)

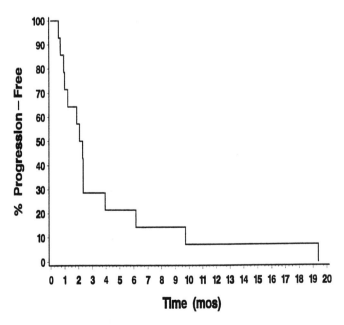

Figure 1   Time to progression.

in Figure 1. Overall survival for the intent-to-treat study group ($n =$ 16) is shown in Figure 2, with a median length of survival of 3.9 months and a 1-year survival of 26%. Included in this analysis is one patient who was felt to have metastatic disease (multiple pulmonary nodules) at study entry but who later, after a response to paclitaxel, went on to resection of a residual lung carcinoma and a hamartoma. This patient was still alive more than 43 months after entry onto the study. Retrospectively, it was felt that the "metastatic disease" most likely represented a second primary non-small-cell lung cancer and a benign lesion. Analysis of overall survival of the study group excluding this patient is represented by Figure 3, with a median survival of 3.9 months and a 1-year survival of 22%. Of the seven patients who entered the study with an ECOG performance status of 2, four

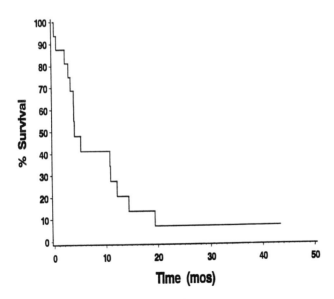

Figure 2   Patient survival (intent-to-treat, $n = 16$).

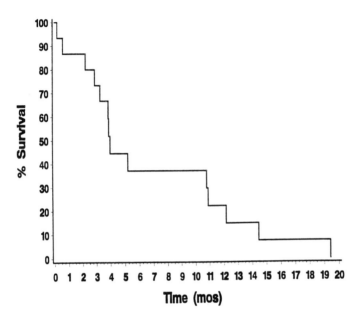

Figure 3 Patient survival ($n = 15$).

had progressive disease. The longest survival in this group of patients was 5.2 months.

DISCUSSION

We performed a retrospective review of patients treated with single-agent, second-line paclitaxel for metastatic NSCLC that had progressed after platinum-based chemotherapy. Disease found in this setting is notoriously refractory to second-line therapy. Paclitaxel showed modest activity and acceptable toxicity in this setting. Hematological toxicity, specifically leukopenia, was frequent but febrile neutropenia was rare. The main nonhematological toxicity was fatigue that appeared to have unique features. It was characterized by a cumulative, profound asthenia that manifested in a subset of patients in a delayed fashion, after several cycles of paclitaxel. It had a substantial impact on patient quality of life, and was dose-limiting for several patients. The pathophysiological mechanism and predisposing factors for this unique toxicity remain elusive. Further investigation may help define ways to abrogate this toxicity in patients receiving paclitaxel.

The response rate reported here is in the range of other second-line therapies. Several of the minor responses were quite prolonged and may reflect inhibition of angiogenesis that has recently been described for paclitaxel (9,10).

Despite a median survival of < 6 months, the 1-year survival of 22% is noteworthy in patients with platinum-resistant NSCLC. These survival statistics should be viewed within the context of the study population, as almost one-half of patients had a relatively poor performance status (ECOG 2). Not surprisingly, these patients did less well than those patients with a performance status of 0 to 1 (8).

As paclitaxel's role as an important first-line agent in combination with platinum compounds continues to be defined, its role as a second-line agent will undoubtedly become more limited. Still, for patients who have disease that has progressed after platinum compounds in combination with other agents, second-line paclitaxel appears to have moderate efficacy and acceptable toxicity. Careful selection of patients for paclitaxel in this setting is warranted, as its use in patients with relatively poor performance status may not be appropriate.

REFERENCES

1. Weick JK, Crowley J, Natale RB, et al. A randomized trial of five cisplatin-containing treatments in patients with metastatic non-small cell lung cancer: a Southwest Oncology Group study. J Clin Oncol 1991; 9:1157–1162.
2. Murphy WK, Fossella F, Winn RJ, et al. Phase II study of Taxol in patients with untreated advanced non-small cell lung cancer. J Natl Cancer Inst 1993; 85:384–388.

3. Chang AY, Kim K, Glick J, et al. Phase II study of Taxol, merbarone, and piroxantrone in stage IV non-small cell lung cancer: The Eastern Cooperative Oncology Group results. J Natl Cancer Inst 1993; 85: 388–394.

4. Ruckdeschel JC, Finkelstein DM, Ettinger DS, et al. A randomized trial of the four most active regimens for metastatic non-small cell lung cancer. J Clin Oncol 1986; 4:14–22.

5. Finkelstein DM, Ettinger DS, Ruckdeschel JC. Long-term survivors in metastatic non-small cell lung cancer: an Eastern Cooperative Oncology Group study. J Clin Oncol 1986; 4:702–709.

6. Kris M, Gralla R, Wertheim M. Trial of the combination of mitomycin, vindesine and cisplatin in patients with advanced non-small cell lung cancer. Cancer Treat Rep 1986; 70:1091–1096.

7. Gralla RJ, Kris MG, Potanovich LM, et al. Enhancing the safety and efficacy of the MVP regimen (mitomycin + vinblastine + cisplatin) in 100 patients with inoperable non-small cell lung cancer. Proc Am Soc Clin Oncol 1989; 8:227. Abstract.

8. Finkelstein DM, Ettinger DS, Ruckdeschel JC. Long-term survivors in metastatic non-small cell lung cancer: an Eastern Cooperative Oncology Group study. J Clin Oncol 1986; 4:702.

9. Belotti D, Nicoletti I, Vergani V, et al. Paclitaxel (Taxol), a microtubule affecting drug, inhibits induced angiogenesis. Proc Annu Meet Am Assoc Cancer Res 1996; 37:397. Abstract.

10. Dordunoo SK, Jackson JK, Arsenault LA, Oktaba AM, Hunter WL, Burt HM. Taxol encapsulation in poly(epsilon-caprolactone) microspheres. Cancer Chemother Pharmacol 1995; 36:279–282.

11

Docetaxel in Chemotherapy-Refractory or Recurrent Non-Small-Cell Lung Cancer

Frank V. Fossella, Jin Soo Lee, and Waun Ki Hong
University of Texas M.D. Anderson Cancer Center, Houston, Texas

INTRODUCTION

The taxane docetaxel (Taxotere) produces a major response rate of 24 to 34% when administered at 100 mg/m^2 over 1 h every 3 weeks as a first-line agent in chemotherapy-naive good-performance-status patients with advanced non-small-cell lung cancer (NSCLC) (1–5). Average median survival in this chemotherapy-naive group of patients is 39 weeks and 1-year survival is 34%. Data from two Phase II trials suggests that docetaxel has activity in the second-line setting as well.

In order to gain an appropriate perspective regarding docetaxel's role in the second-line treatment of NSCLC, however, one must first have a good understanding of the issues surrounding the relative benefits of chemotherapy in the first-line setting. Advanced NSCLC (i.e., inoperable tumors for which one would not consider an aggressive chemoradiation approach) remains a relatively chemotherapy-resistant tumor that is essentially incurable, even in a best-case scenario of the "good-prognosis" patient (i.e., healthy, good performance status, with minimal weight loss) receiving first-line treatment. Thus, the relative benefits of chemotherapy versus palliative care only, even in a front-line setting, are debatable. Randomized studies comparing cisplatin-based combination chemotherapy to best supportive care for advanced NSCLC has shown only a minor (though statistically significant) impact on survival: median survival improved from 17 weeks to 27 weeks, and 1-year survival increased from 5 to 15% in patients who received chemotherapy (6,7).

Despite the marginal benefit of chemotherapy for this disease, most medical oncologists feel that it is reasonable at least to offer a trial of front-line systemic chemotherapy, usually with a platinum-based combination regimen, to patients with advanced NSCLC who have an acceptable performance status (i.e., 0 or 1, and possibly 2), who are otherwise in good health, and who understand that the positive impact of therapy on quality of life and/or survival may be marginal.

Given the fact that the benefits of first-line platinum-based chemotherapy for advanced NSCLC may be minimal, the indications for second-line treatment of the patient who has failed initial chemotherapy are even more debatable. Not only do these patients generally have a worse performance status than the chemotherapy-naive patient, but intuitively we might expect these patients to have tumors refractory to all chemotherapy due to an inherent and/or acquired drug resistance. Nonetheless, such patients often do request of their medical oncologist a trial of second-line therapy, and we need to develop rational and cost-effective guidelines to follow in this setting.

CLINICAL TRIALS OF DOCETAXEL AS
SECOND-LINE THERAPY FOR NSCLC

There are few chemotherapy drugs whose second-line efficacy against NSCLC has been specifically or systematically evaluated. The exception is docetaxel, whose activity as a second-line agent in patients with platinum-resistant or refractory NSCLC has been extensively studied in two large Phase II trials and in two ongoing randomized Phase III trials.

Phase II Studies of Second-Line Docetaxel for NSCLC

The two Phase II studies were identical protocols which accrued a total of 88 patients. They were conducted at M.D. Anderson Cancer Center (MDACC) (44 patients) and University of Texas at San Antonio (UTSA) (44 patients, enrolled at three sites) (4,5,8,9).

Eligible patients had stage IV or unresectable stage III NSCLC, a life expectancy of at least 12 weeks, and a performance status of $\leq$ 2 (Zubrod's scale). Patients must have received and failed at least one prior chemotherapy regimen containing cisplatin and/or carboplatin; patients who had received more than two prior regimens were ineligible. "Platinum-resistant" patients were defined as those whose disease showed an initial response to a platinum-containing regimen (either complete/partial response or stable disease) but then subsequently progressed; "platinum-refractory" patients were those whose disease never showed response to platinum-containing chemotherapy. The starting dose of docetaxel was 100 mg/m^2 as a 1-h infusion every 21 days.

Eighty-eight patients were enrolled in these two studies: 46 men and 42 women, with a median age of 57 (range, 29 to 77). It is important to note that most patients had a very good performance status (0 or 1 in 86%) despite their advanced disease and extensive prior therapy. Sixteen percent of patients had stage III disease and 84% had stage IV. Most patients had adenocarcinoma (65%), and 56% had received prior radiotherapy. Using the definitions described above, 58% of patients were platinum-resistant and 42% were platinum-refractory (Table 1).

Fourteen of 71 evaluable patients (19.7%) achieved a partial response to treatment; the response rate in the intent-to-treat population was 17% (95% CI 9.9 to 26.6%) (Table 2). There was a trend to more responses in patients with adenocarcinoma versus nonadenocarcinoma, but this was not statistically significant. In the MDACC study there was no difference in response rate between the patients who were platinum-resistant versus platinum-refractory. Median time

Table 1 Patient Characteristics: Platinum-Refractory/
Resistant Patients Treated with Docetaxel 100 mg/m^2
Every 3 Weeks

	No. of patients
Patients entered	88
MDACC	44
UTSA	44[a]
Median age (range), years	57 (29–77)
Gender	
Men	46 (52%)
Women	42 (48%)
Stage	
III	14 (16%)
IV	74 (84%)
Performance status	
0/1	75 (86%)
2	13 (14%)
Histology	
Adenocarcinoma	57 (65%)
Squamous carcinoma	15 (17%)
Adenosquamous	1 (1%)
Large-cell carcinoma	11 (13%)
Unclassified non-small-cell	4 (5%)
Previous therapy	
Surgery	27 (31%)
Radiotherapy	49 (56%)
Chemotherapy	88 (100%)
Platinum-resistant	51 (58%)
Platinum-refractory	37 (42%)

Source: Ref. 5.
[a]Accrued at three sites.

to partial response was 6 weeks (or two courses of treatment). The
median duration of response was 29 weeks (range, 17+ to 46+ weeks),
and median time to progression was 14 weeks. The projected median
survival (both studies, all patients) is 39 weeks (95% CI: 33.3 to 52.8
weeks), and projected 1-year survival is 40% (Fig. 1).

Table 2 Response to Treatment: Platinum-Refractory/Resistant Patients Treated with Docetaxel 100 mg/m^2 Every 3 Weeks

Institution	Partial response (evaluable patients)	Partial response (intent-to-treat)	Median response duration (wk)	Median survival (mo)
MDACC	8/36 (22.2%) (95% CI: 10%–39%)	9/44 (20.5%) (95% CI: 10–35%)	30	11
UTSA[a]	6/35 (17.1%) (95% CI: 7%–34%)	6/44 (13.6%) (95% CI: 5%–27%)	26	5.8
Total	14/71 (19.7%)	15/88 (17.0%) (95% CI: 10%–27%)	29	9 (95% CI: 8–12)

Source: Ref. 5.
[a]Accrued at 3 sites.

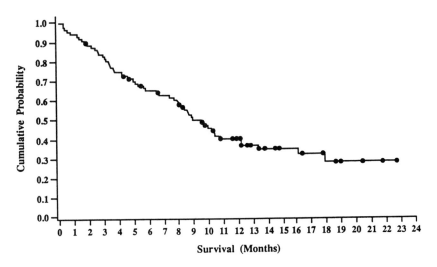

Figure 1 Projected survival (88 patients, two studies) of platinum-refractory/resistant patients with advanced non-small-cell lung cancer treated with docetaxel (all patients). (From Ref. 5.)

We noted that the patients in the MDACC group showed a higher response rate (21% versus 14%) and median survival (42 weeks versus 25 weeks) than those at UTSA. This could be explained by the fact that only 2/44 patients (5%) in the MDACC cohort had a performance status 2 versus 10/44 patients (23%) at UTSA.

Comparison of Docetaxel Phase II Data with Historical Controls

The survival outcome of these trials compares favorably with that of historical controls as determined in a retrospective review undertaken at MDACC (10). For that analysis we screened our computerized protocol data management base and identified a cohort of 36 patients with advanced NSCLC who were enrolled on a variety of Phase I studies at MDACC after having failed standard front-line combination chemotherapy (platinum-based in all but one patient). We considered this cohort an appropriate comparison arm because these were patients who would otherwise have been eligible for our second-line docetaxel study had that protocol been active at the time. Furthermore, because these patients were enrolled in other clinical trials at our institution, we had reliable prospective data regarding key patient characteristics, long-term follow-up, and survival.

Both the docetaxel group ($n = 44$) and the historical controls ($n = 36$) were well balanced with regard to age, gender, stage, histology, number of prior chemotherapy cycles, and response to front-line combination chemotherapy. One significant difference between the two groups was a greater preponderance of patients with performance status of 2 in the historical controls (7/36 patients, or 19%) compared with the docetaxel patients (2/44, or 5%) (Table 3).

Partial responses were seen in 9/44 patients (21%) treated with docetaxel; no major responses were seen in the control patients receiving Phase I therapies. Recently updated survival data show a median survival (all patients) of 41 weeks for the docetaxel patients ($n = 44$) versus 16 weeks for the historical control group ($n = 36$), and 1-year survival of 39% (docetaxel) versus 16% (controls); this was statistically significant ($p = .003$) (Fig. 2). We also performed a Kaplan-Meier survival analysis for the good-performance-status (i.e., 0 or 1)

Table 3 Patient Characteristics and Results: MDACC Patients Treated with Second-Line Docetaxel Versus Historical Controls

	Docetaxel ($n = 44$)	Historical control ($n = 36$)
Age: median/range	57/29–71	55 (37–74)
Male/female	26/18	22/14
Stage		
IIIb	4 (9%)	4 (11%)
IV	40 (91%)	32 (89%)
PS		
0/1	42 (95%)	29 (81%)
2	2 (5%)	7 (19%)
Histology		
Adenocarcinoma	27 (61%)	24 (67%)
Squamous	7 (16%)	7 (19%)
Large cell	5 (11%)	0
Adenosquamous	1 (2%)	0
Unclassified NSC	4 (9%)	5 (14%)
Prior chemotherapy		
1 regimen	26 (59%)	32 (89%)
2 regimens	18 (41%)	4 (11%)
< 6 cycles	31 (70%)	27 (75%)
≥ 6 cycles	13 (30%)	9 (25%)
Response to primary chemotherapy		
Yes	7 (16%)	5 (14%)
No	36 (82%)	20 (83%)
Unknown	1 (2%)	1 (3%)
PR to study drug	9 (21%)	0
Survival (all patients)		
Median	42 weeks	16 weeks
1-year	41%	16%
Survival (PS 0/1 patients)		
Median	43 weeks	16 weeks
1-year	42%	16%

Source: Ref. 10.
Abbreviations: PS, Zubrod performance status; NSC, non-small-cell carcinoma; PR, partial response.

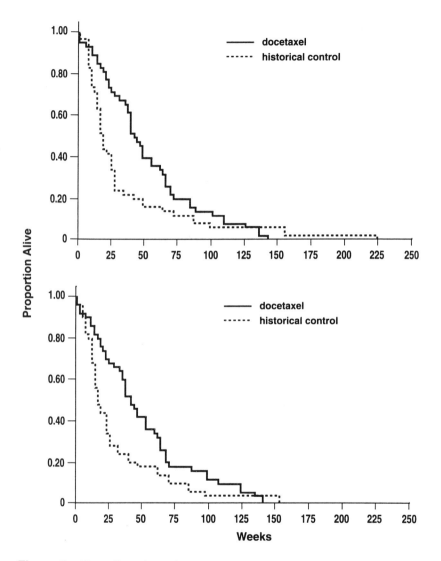

Figure 2 Overall projected survival of patients treated with second-line docetaxel versus historical controls: all patients (top panel; $p = .003$), and patients with performance status 0/1 (bottom panel; $p = .018$). (From Ref. 10.)

patients only, since the control group had more patients of perform-ance status 2 which might have skewed the survival in favor of the docetaxel arm. That analysis also showed a statistically significant improvement in survival for the docetaxel patients: median and 1-year survivals were 43 weeks and 42% ($n = 42$) versus 16 weeks and 16% for the 29 historical controls ($p = .018$) (Fig. 2). It should be noted that the 16-week median and 16% 1-year survivals noted in our control arm were equivalent to those reported for the "best sup-portive care" arm of numerous studies comparing front-line chemo-therapy to best supportive care; this tends to support the validity of having selected this group as an appropriate comparator (6,7).

Phase III Studies of Second-Line Docetaxel for NSCLC

Despite the obvious limitations of this retrospective analysis, it does provide some insight into the relative survival advantage of using docetaxel as second-line treatment for patients who have failed first-line platinum-based chemotherapy. This issue will be more directly addressed by two large ongoing randomized studies of good per-formance status patients with advanced NSCLC whose disease has failed to respond to at least one prior platinum-containing regimen. In the first study patients are randomized between docetaxel 100 mg/m^2 intravenously over 1 h every 21 days or best supportive care. The second study randomizes patients between docetaxel 100 mg/m^2 versus docetaxel 75 mg/m^2 versus a third "control arm" of either vi-norelbine or ifosfamide. The primary endpoint of both studies is sur-vival; secondary endpoints are quality of life, response rate, and tox-icity. These studies are ongoing, and preliminary results should be available soon.

OTHER AGENTS AS SECOND-LINE THERAPY FOR REFRACTORY NSCLC

The related taxane, paclitaxel (Taxol), has not been as systematically studied in the second-line setting, and available data are conflicting. While one trial suggests that paclitaxel at 200 mg/m^2 over 1 h produces a respectable response rate in platinum-resistant patients (11), the cohort of patients studied was small and survival data are unavailable. In contrast, five other small studies have reported no or minimal second-line activity with paclitaxel (although there was a greater proportion of performance-status 2 patients enrolled in these trials than in the two large docetaxel studies discussed, which may have affected results) (12–16). The available data on other drugs, including vinorelbine (17–19), CPT-11 (20–22), vindesine (23–28), and mitomycin (29–31), have been similarly disappointing.

CONCLUSION

In conclusion, two large Phase II studies have demonstrated that docetaxel at 100 mg/m^2 every 21 days has some activity against platinum-resistant/refractory NSCLC. A comparison of survival data from one of those trials with historical controls suggests, furthermore, that there may be a clinically meaningful survival advantage of docetaxel in this setting as well: 16 weeks versus 42 weeks median, and 16% versus 41% at 1 year. It must be stressed, however, that most patients in these studies (particularly the one conducted at MDACC) were of excellent performance status despite their extensive prior therapy. Two large ongoing randomized trials comparing docetaxel to either best supportive care or to other active agents will better define this drug's role in the second-line treatment for NSCLC. The available information regarding the second-line activity of other agents is scanty and has been rather disappointing.

Given these data and pending the results of larger randomized trials, a reasonable practice at this time would be to offer a trial of second-line chemotherapy with docetaxel (and perhaps paclitaxel) to patients with NSCLC who have failed first-line platinum-based treatment. However, because most of the subjects enrolled in the positive trials were in very good condition, the use of second-line taxane therapy in a nonprotocol setting should probably be limited as well to good-performance-status patients (i.e., 0 or 1), particularly since we know that there is little, if any, benefit of front-line chemotherapy in poor-performance-status patients.

REFERENCES

1. Fossella FV, Lee JS, Murphy WK, et al. Phase II study of docetaxel for recurrent or metastatic non-small cell lung cancer. J Clin Oncol 1994; 12:1238–1244.
2. Francis PA,Rigas JR, Kris MG, et al. Phase II trial of docetaxel in patients with stage III and IV non-small cell lung cancer. J Clin Oncol 1994; 12:1232–1237.
3. Cerny T, Kaplan S, Pavlidis N, et al. Docetaxel (Taxotere) is active in non-small cell lung cancer: a phase II trial of the EORTC early clinical trials group (ECTG). Br J Cancer 1994; 70:384–387.
4. Burris HA, Eckardt J, Fields S, et al. Phase II trials of Taxotere in patients with non-small cell lung cancer. Proc Am Soc Clin Oncol 1993; 12:335. Abstract.
5. Fossella FV, Lee JS, Berille J, et al. Summary of phase II data of docetaxel (Taxotere), an active agent in the first- and second-line treatment of advanced non-small cell lung cancer. Semin Oncol 1995; 22 (suppl 4):22–29.
6. Non-Small Cell Lung Cancer Collaborative Group. Chemotherapy in non-small cell lung cancer: a meta-analysis using updated data on individual patients from 52 randomised clinical trials. Br Med J 1995; 311:899–909.
7. Grilli R, Oxman AD, Julian JA. Chemotherapy for advanced non-small cell lung cancer: how much benefit is enough? J Clin Oncol 1993; 11: 1866–1872.
8. Fossella FV, Lee JS, Shin DM, et al. Phase II study of docetaxel for advanced or metastatic platinum-refractory non-small cell lung cancer. J Clin Oncol 1995; 13:645–651.
9. Rhône-Poulenc Rorer. Taxotere (docetaxel) presentation to the Oncology Drugs Advisory Committee of the Federal Drug Administration; Rockville, MD; Dec. 13, 1994.
10. Fossella FV, Lee JS. Docetaxel for platinum-refractory non-small cell lung cancer: comparison of phase II results to historical controls. Unpublished data.
11. Hainsworth JD, Thompson DA, Greco FA. Paclitaxel by 1-hour infusion: an active drug in metastatic non-small cell lung cancer. J Clin Oncol 1995; 13:1609–1614.
12. Murphy WK, Winn RJ, Huber M, et al. Phase II study of Taxol in patients with non-small cell lung cancer who have failed platinum containing chemotherapy. Proc Am Soc Clin Oncol 1994; 13:363. Abstract.

13. Roa V, Conner A, Mitchell RB. Carboplatin and paclitaxel for advanced non-small cell lung cancer in previously treated patients. Proc Am Soc Clin Oncol 1996; 15:403. Abstract.

14. Stewart DJ, Tomiak E, Goss G, et al. Paclitaxel plus low dose hydroxyurea as second line therapy in non-small cell lung cancer. Proc Am Soc Clin Oncol 1995; 14:367. Abstract.

15. Tan V, Herrera C, Einzig AI, et al. Taxol is active as a 3 hour or 24 hour infusion in non-small cell lung cancer. Proc Am Soc Clin Oncol 1995; 14:366. Abstract.

16. Ruckdeschel J, Wagner H, Williams C, ct al. Second-line chemotherapy for resistant metastatic non-small cell lung cancer: the role of Taxol. Proc Am Soc Clin Oncol 1994; 13:357. Abstract.

17. Pronzato P, Landucci M, Vaira F, et al. Failure of vinorelbine to produce responses in pretreated non-small cell lung cancer patients. Anticancer Res 1994; 14:1413–1416.

18. Rinaldi M, Della Giulia M, Venturo I, et al. Vinorelbine as single agent in the treatment of advanced non-small cell lung cancer. Proc Am Soc Clin Oncol 1994; 13:360. Abstract.

19. Santoro A, Maiorino L, Santoro M. Second-line with vinorelbine in the weekly monochemotherapy for the treatment of advanced non-small cell lung cancer. Lung Cancer 1994; 11(suppl 1):130. Abstract.

20. CPT-11 Cooperative Study Group. A phase II study of CPT-11, a camptothecin derivative, in patients with primary lung cancer. Jpn J Cancer Chemother 1991; 18:1013–1019.

21. Nakai H, Fukuoka M, Furuse K, et al. An early phase II study of CPT-11 for primary lung cancer. Jpn J Cancer Chemother 1991; 18:607–612.

22. Niitani H, Fukuoka M, Nagao K. Clinical development of irinotecan (CPT-11) in lung cancers. Lung Cancer 1994; 11(suppl 2):30–31.

23. Sculier JP, Bureau G, Thiriaux J, et al. High dose epirubicin (120 mg/m^2) plus vindesine is not an effective salvage regimen for advanced non-small cell lung cancer priorly treated with a cisplatin containing regimen. Ann Oncol 1994; 5(suppl 8):159. Abstract.

24. Gridelli C, Airoma G, Incoronato P, et al. Mitomycin C plus vindesine or cisplatin plus epirubicin in previously treated patients with symptomatic advanced non-small cell lung cancer. Cancer Chemother Pharmacol 1992; 30:212–214.

25. Fuks JZ, Egorin MJ, Aisner J, et al. Therapeutic efficacy and pharmacokinetics of vindesine and vindesine-cisplatin in previously treated patients with non-small cell lung carcinoma. Cancer Chemother Pharmacol 1983; 10:104–108.

26. Gralla RJ, Raphael BG, Golbey RB, et al. Phase II evaluation of vindesine in patients with non-small cell carcinoma of the lung. Cancer Treat Rep 1979; 63:1343–1346.

27. Furnas BE, Williams SD, Einhorn LH, et al. Vindesine: an effective agent in the treatment of non-small cell lung cancer. Cancer Treat Rep 1982; 66:1709–1711.

28. Luedke SL, Luedke DW, Petruska P, et al. Vindesine monochemotherapy for non-small cell lung cancer: a report of 45 cases. Cancer Treat Rep 1982; 66:1409–1411.

29. Bonomi PD, Finkelstein DM, Ruckdeschel JC, et al. Combination chemotherapy versus single agents followed by combination chemotherapy in stage IV non-small cell lung cancer: a study of the Eastern Cooperative Oncology Group. J Clin Oncol 1989; 7:1602–1613.

30. Dansin E, Sokpoh H, Georges H, et al. Mitomycin, ifosfamide, cisplatin (MIC) as second-line regimen in advanced non-small cell lung cancer. Ann Oncol 1992; 3(suppl 5):35. Abstract.

31. Bervar JF, Durieu J, Brichet A, et al. MIC (mitomycin C, ifosfamide, cisplatin) as a second line treatment for non-small cell lung carcinomas. Ann Oncol 1994; 5(suppl 8):152. Abstract.

12

Paclitaxel

Combinations with Cisplatin or Carboplatin
in Non-Small-Cell Lung Cancer

Chandra P. Belani
*University of Pittsburgh School of Medicine and University of
Pittsburgh Cancer Institute, Pittsburgh, Pennsylvania*

INTRODUCTION

Paclitaxel, a novel diterpene plant product, identified initially as the active constituent in the bark of the Pacific yew tree, *Taxus brevefolia*, is now obtained via a semisynthetic process. It is one of the unique antimicrotubule agents that shifts the equilibrium toward microtubule assembly and stabilizes tubulin polymer formation. This disrupts the normal dynamic reorganization of the microtubule network essential for vital interphase and mitotic function (1,2). It has demonstrated promising activity in early trials in non-small-cell lung cancer (NSCLC) (3–6). A randomized Phase II Eastern Cooperative Oncology Group (ECOG) trial of paclitaxel (250 mg/m^2, 24-h infusion every 3 weeks) and other investigational agents (merbarone and piroxantrone) yielded an overall response rate of 21% in patients with metastatic NSCLC, with a 1-year survival of 41% (4). The ECOG investigators concluded that paclitaxel was the most active agent evaluated by the group against NSCLC. These results were confirmed in a similar Phase II trial of paclitaxel (200 mg/m^2, 24-h infusion every 3 weeks) conducted at the M.D. Anderson Cancer Center. Due to initial concerns of hypersensitivity reactions with paclitaxel (cremophor vehicle), early studies used paclitaxel at 24-h infusion schedules (3,4). These have been substantially reduced with the use of premedications which include dexamethasone, diphenhydramine, and H$_2$-blocking agents (1,7).

Shorter infusion schedules (3-h and 1-h) offer the advantage of avoiding hospitalization and, when used with the standard premedications, do not appear to increase the occurrence of hypersensitivity reactions (6,8,9). The 3-h paclitaxel infusion schedule studied by Gatzmeier et al., at the dose of 225 mg/m^2 every 3 weeks, resulted in a 24% response rate in patients with Stage III B and Stage IV NSCLC, and the median survival was 10 months (5). The response rate in NSCLC with paclitaxel 175 mg/m^2 over 3 h was lower (10%) in the Australian study (6), but the 1-year survival was again 40%, leading to further confirmation of its activity when administered at short-infusion schedules. Same degree of activity has been observed with paclitaxel administered at 1-h infusion schedule in patients with advanced NSCLC (9,10). For future studies paclitaxel doses of 200 to 225 mg/m^2 appear to be well tolerated and are feasible using 3-h or 1-h infusion allowing greater ease of administration in an outpatient setting.

PACLITAXEL-CISPLATIN COMBINATION IN NSCLC

Paclitaxel, when used in combination with cisplatin, demonstrates a sequence-dependent drug interaction (11,12). There is an increase in myelotoxicity, i.e., neutropenia, when cisplatin is administered prior to paclitaxel. This is probably due to the effect of cisplatin on cytochrome P-450 enzymes, resulting in decreased plasma clearance of paclitaxel (13). Thus it is recommended that the sequence of administration be in the order of paclitaxel followed by cisplatin when the two drugs are used in combination.

The paclitaxel-cisplatin combination has been evaluated in three small Phase I-II studies (14–16) in NSCLC. The activity in advanced NSCLC has ranged from 35% to 47% (Table 1). In the study reported by Klastersky et al. (14), 17 patients were treated with cisplatin 100 mg/m^2 in combination with paclitaxel doses ranging from 135 mg/m^2 to 200 mg/m^2 (3-h infusion). The response rate in this study was 47% but the treatment had to be discontinued in five patients after three courses of therapy due to development of severe polyneuropathy (14). The combination pf paclitaxel-cisplatin is active in NSCLC, but is associated with neuropathy which is both dose-related and cumulative. To further evaluate the paclitaxel-cisplatin regimen in advanced NSCLC and also to study the dose-response effect with paclitaxel in NSCLC, ECOG mounted a large Phase III trial (17) comparing etoposide-cisplatin combination with high dose (250 mg/m^2 with granulocyte colony-stimulating factor) or modest dose (135 mg/m^2) paclitaxel in combination with cisplatin (75 mg/m^2) (Table 2). Paclitaxel was administered on both the high-dose and modest-dose arms on a 24-h infusion schedule, and cycles were repeated every 3 weeks. The response rates for the modest-dose and high-dose paclitaxel arms observed were 26.5% and 32.1%, respectively, showing significant benefit ($p < .001$) when compared to the etoposide-cisplatin arm (12%). The 1-year survival rates for the paclitaxel-cisplatin arms were 36.9% (modest-dose paclitaxel) and 39.1% (high-dose paclitaxel), showing a trend toward longer survival compared to the etoposide-cisplatin regimen which resulted in a 1-year survival of 31.6%. Based on the results of this study, ECOG has adopted paclitaxel (135 mg/m^2, 24-h infusion) in combination with cisplatin (75 mg/m^2) with cycles repeated every 3 weeks as the new reference regimen for future randomized trials in NSCLC, replacing the etoposide-cisplatin regimen.

Paclitaxel administered either biweekly (18) or as a prolonged 4-day infusion (19) has been tested in combination with cisplatin against NSCLC, and the preliminary results show that these regimens are feasible but require further study (Table 3).

PACLITAXEL AND CARBOPLATIN COMBINATION IN NSCLC

Carboplatin, developed as a less toxic analog of its parent cisplatin (20,21), had shown marginal activity against NSCLC in terms of

Table 1 Paclitaxel (3-h infusion) and Cisplatin: Phase I-II Studies

Authors	Schema	Number of patients	Response rate	Median survival (months)	1 year survival	Comments
Klastersky et al. (14)	Paclitaxel 135–200 mg/m^2 Cisplatin 100 mg/m^2	17	47%	—	—	Severe late neurological toxicity in 5 patients
Pirker et al. (15)	Paclitaxel 175 mg/m^2 Cisplatin 100 mg/m^2	20	35%	10	35%	Neuropathy was significant
Belli et al. (16)	Paclitaxel 135–225 mg/m^2 Cisplatin 100–120 mg/m^2	29	38%	—	—	—

Table 2 The Eastern Cooperative Oncology Group (ECOG) Phase III Randomized Comparison of Cisplatin-Etoposide vs. Cisplatin-Paclitaxel (modest dose) vs. Cisplatin-Paclitaxel (high dose) with Filgrastim Support for Patients with Advanced and Metastatic NSCLC

Study	Scheme	Patients	Response rate	Median survival (months)	1-year survival
ECOG (17)	Arm A Paclitaxel (24-h infusion) 135 mg/m^2 and cisplatin 75 mg/m^2		26.5%	9.56	36.9%
	Arm B Paclitaxel (24-h infusion) 250 mg/m^2 and cisplatin 75 mg/m^2 (+ G-CSF)	560 (in all 3 arms)	32.1%	9.99	39.1%
	Arm C Etoposide 100 mg/m^2, days 1–3, cisplatin 75 mg/m^2		12.0%	7.69	31.6%
	(cycles repeated every 3 weeks)				

Table 3 Paclitaxel (biweekly and 4-day infusion) and Cisplatin: Early Results of Phase I-II Studies

Authors	Schema	Cycle duration	Number of patients	Response rate	Comments
Gelmon et al. (18)	Paclitaxel (3-h) 100 mg/m^2 → 140 mg/m^2 Cisplatin 60 mg/m^2	2 weeks	16	56%	Maximum tolerated dose not reached. Well-tolerated biweekly regimen.
Georgiadis et al. (19)	Paclitaxel 100 → 140 mg/m^2 4-day infusion Cisplatin 60–80 mg/m^2	3–4 weeks	16	56%	Maximum tolerated dose without filgrastim support is paclitaxel 120 mg/m^2 4-day infusion and cisplatin 80 mg/m^2

response rates (22,23). However, when the combination of carbo-platin and etoposide was compared to the cisplatin-etoposide regimen in a randomized trial for patients with advanced and metastatic NSCLC, there was no significant difference in either activity or survival between the two arms (24). The carboplatin-etoposide regimen had a favorable toxicity profile, producing significantly less leukopenia, nausea, and vomiting and diarrhea than the cisplatin-etoposide combination. Carboplatin, when compared to three cisplatin-based combination regimens in a randomized ECOG study (22) for patients with Stage IV NSCLC, yielded superior survival and less toxicity. Carboplatin, with thrombocytopenia as its dose-limiting toxicity, was thus a suitable agent to combine with paclitaxel.

The paclitaxel-carboplatin regimen has been tested by a number of investigators in advanced and metastatic NSCLC (Tables 3–5) (25–36), and the results have been promising. The early studies used the 24-h infusion schedule of paclitaxel in combination with carboplatin (25–27). In our Phase I metastatic NSCLC study of this combination (25), the dose of paclitaxel was initially fixed at 135 mg/m^2 given as a 24-h infusion with carboplatin administered in escalating doses based on a target area under the concentration time curve (AUC) of 5, 7, 9 or 11 using Calvert's formula: Dose (mg) = (Glomerular filtration rate [GFR] + 25). The GFR was substituted by a measured 24-h urinary creatinine clearance. Grade 4 thrombocytopenia was dose-limiting at carboplatin dose targeted to achieve an AUC of 11 mg/ml·min. The paclitaxel dose was then escalated to 175 mg/m^2, 200 mg/m^2, and 225 mg/m^2 in cohorts. Rare nonhematological toxicities included fatigue, diarrhea, and nausea and vomiting. Among the first 30 patients, one had a complete response and 14 had partial responses for an overall response rate of 50%. The recommended doses for future studies were paclitaxel 175 mg/m^2 (24-h infusion) without granulocyte-colony stimulating factor (G-CSF) or 225 mg/m^2 (24-h infusion) with G-CSF in combination with carboplatin dose based on an AUC of 7 mg/ml·min. Myeloprotective effect of paclitaxel on carboplatin-associated thrombocytopenia was demonstrated by the results of this study when comparisons were made on the effect of percent decreases in platelets with the combination of paclitaxel and carboplatin versus carboplatin alone from historical data (37).

Table 4 Paclitaxel (24-h infusion) and Carboplatin: Phase I-II Studies in Advanced and Metastatic NSCLC

Authors	Paclitaxel dose (mg/m²)	Carboplatin dose	Cycle duration (weeks)	# Patients	RR[a]	Median survival (weeks)	1-yr survival	Comments
Belani et al. (25)	135, 175, 200, 225 mg/m²	AUC = 5, 7, 9, 11 mg/ml·min	3	36	50%	—	—	Recommended doses: paclitaxel 175 mg/m² with carboplatin AUC = 7 without G-CSF and paclitaxel 225 mg/m² with cisplatin AUC=7 with G-CSF support
Langer et al. (26)	135→215 mg/m² (intrapatient escalation)	AUC=7.5 mg/ml·min	3	53	62%	53	54%	Myelosuppression principal toxicity Paclitaxel dose to 215 mg/m² in ≥ 70% patients who received 3 or more cycles
Johnson et al. (27)	135 mg/m²	300 mg/m²	4	16	18%	33		Women lived longer than men (53.7 vs. 31.2 wk)
	135 mg/m²	AUC = 6 mg/ml·min	4	12			32% all patients	
	175 mg/m²	AUC = 6 mg/ml·min	4	23	39%	38		Suggestion of dose-response effect with paclitaxel

[a]RR = response rate.

Table 5 Paclitaxel (3-h infusion) and Carboplatin: Phase I-II Studies in Advanced and Metastatic NSCLC

Authors	Paclitaxel dose (mg/m^2)	Carboplatin dose	Cycle duration (weeks)	Number of patients	Response rate	Comments
Natale et al. (28)	150 → 250	AUC = 6 (mg/ml·min)	3	42	62%	Recommended doses: paclitaxel 225 mg/m^2 3-h infusion with carboplatin dose calculated to achieve AUC = 6 mg/ml·min
Rowinsky et al. (29)	175 → 225	AUC 7/9 (mg/ml·min)	3	19	37%	Recommended doses: paclitaxel 225 mg/m^2 with carboplatin AUC = 7 mg/ml·min
Schutte et al. (30)	200	AUC = 5 (mg/ml·min)	3	25	52%	Active regimen myalgia (48%) and neuropathy (48%) were the most common side effects
Bunn et al. (31)	135	250–350 mg/m^2	3	12	8%	Suggestion of dose-response effect with paclitaxel in combination with carboplatin
	175	350–400 mg/m^2	3	9	33%	
	200	400 mg/m^2	3	7	43%	
Giaccone et al. (32)	100–175	300–400 mg/m^2	4	19	5%	Late responses observed. No sequence-dependent pharmacodynamic effects
	≥175–250	300–400 mg/m^2	4	30	20%	

In the study (26) performed at the Fox Chase Cancer Center and affiliated hospitals, patients with Stage IIIB and IV NSCLC were treated with carboplatin dose targeted to achieve an AUC of 7.5 mg/ml·min in combination with paclitaxel dose (24-h infusion) escalated from 135 mg/m^2 to 175 and then 215 mg/m^2 intrapatient with subsequent cycles. By the sixth cycle, 30% of patients had grade 3/4 thrombocytopenia, 31% had myalgias and arthralgias, and 38% had neurotoxicity (therapy discontinued in only one patient secondary to neuropathy). Paclitaxel dose was escalated to 215 mg/m^2 in $\geq 70\%$ of patients who received three or more cycles. The overall response rate was 62%, with a complete response rate of 9%. The median survival was 53 weeks and the 1-year survival was 54%. These intriguing results are by far the best reported in the literature.

A suggestion of dose-response effect with paclitaxel in NSCLC, when used in combination with carboplatin, was seen with most of the responses when the dose of paclitaxel was escalated to ≥ 175 mg/m^2 (27,31). The results from the study by Johnson et al. (27) showed an increase in response rate from 18 to 39% with escalation of the paclitaxel dose from 135 mg/m^2 to 175 mg/m^2 in combination with carboplatin (Table 4). The study also indicated that conventional body surface area dosing of carboplatin results in unpredictable myelosuppression. When the carboplatin dose in the combination was derived using Calvert's formula with a target AUC and calculated GFR, considerable favorable toxicity profile was demonstrated and the dose of paclitaxel could be further escalated. This further validates the importance of pharmacokinetically derived formulas to dose carboplatin in order to obtain an overall improved therapeutic index.

As the optimal schedule of paclitaxel infusion in the combination remained undefined and there was substantial evidence of activity with single agent paclitaxel administered as 3-h infusion, as described earlier (5,6), a number of studies were designed to look at short infusion schedules of paclitaxel with ease of outpatient administration in combination with carboplatin (28–36). The results of these studies are summarized in Tables 5 and 6. Natale (28) escalated the dose of paclitaxel from 150 mg/m^2 to 250 mg/m^2 with increments of 5 mg/m^2 in combination with fixed dose of carboplatin based on a target AUC of 6 mg/ml·min. Dose-limiting toxicities in this study

Table 6 Paclitaxel (1-h) and Carboplatin: Phase I-II Studies in Advanced and Metastatic NSCLC

Authors	Paclitaxel dose	Carboplatin dose	Cycle duration	Number of patients	Response rate	Comments
Hainsworth et al. (33)	225 mg/m²	AUC = 6 mg/ml·min	3 weeks	50	46%	Active regimen
Langer et al. (34)	175 → 280 mg/m² (intrapatient) dose escalation	AUC = 7.5 mg/ml·min	3 weeks	22	55%	Cumulative sensory neuropathy prompting reduction of paclitaxel dose to 135 mg/m² → 215 mg/m²
Roa et al. (35)	200 mg/m²	AUC = 6 mg/ml·min	3 weeks	14	50%	Infusion duration 1–3 h Sensory neuropathy most common non-hematological toxicity
Evans et al. (36)	175 mg/m²	AUC = 6 mg/ml·min	4 weeks → 3 weeks	17 (11 evalu-able)	36%	

were osteoarthralgias/myalgias, cumulative sensory neuropathy, and grade 4 neutropenia. The objective response rate was 62% in the 42 patients with measurable disease. The recommended dose of paclitaxel was 225 mg/m^2, 3-h infusion in combination with carboplatin dose targeted to achieve an AUC of 6 mg/ml·min with cycles repeated every 3 weeks.

In the study of paclitaxel and carboplatin combination for patients with NSCLC reported by Bunn and Kelly (31) paclitaxel was given on a 3-h infusion in doses ranging from 135 to 200 mg/m^2 and carboplatin from 250 to 400 mg/m^2 with cycles repeated every 3 weeks. There was again a suggestion of a dose-response effect against NSCLC with paclitaxel 3-h infusion in this combination, similar to what was seen by Johnson et al. (27). The Dutch study (32) also demonstrated a dose-response effect with short (3-h) infusion of paclitaxel (with carboplatin) in NSCLC. The influence of drug sequence (carboplatin followed by paclitaxel versus paclitaxel followed by carboplatin) does not appear to alter the toxicity and there is no effect of carboplatin on pharmacokinetics of paclitaxel (32), but there is some evidence from in vitro studies (38) that the sequence associated with maximal antitumor efficacy is paclitaxel followed by carboplatin as has been used in most of these studies. The efficacy of the regimen for patients with advanced and metastatic NSCLC appears to be preserved when the paclitaxel infusion duration is decreased to 1 h (33–36) in combination with carboplatin (Table 5).

Thus, short infusion schedules (3 h and 1 h) of paclitaxel have similar degrees of efficacy as compared to 24-h infusion schedules when combined with carboplatin. The dose-limiting toxicity seen with 24-h infusion schedules of paclitaxel in combination with carboplatin is myelosuppression, while shorter infusion schedules (3 h and 1 h) of paclitaxel result in less myelosuppression, but neuropathy and osteoarthralgias/myalgias become dose-limiting. In addition, significant platelet toxicity has not been observed with the paclitaxel/carboplatin combination, and there is a suggestion that paclitaxel may protect against the thrombocytopenia induced by carboplatin, probably because of its unique antimicrotubule effects (37). Dose-response effect with paclitaxel (in combination with carboplatin) against NSCLC has been demonstrated both with 24-h and

3-h infusion schedules with most of the responses seen when the dose of paclitaxel is escalated to ≥ 175 mg/m^2. Full doses of both the agents have been combined without any apparent increase in toxicity (25–28,29,34). Conventional body surface area dosing of carboplatin results in unpredictable myelosuppression, lending further support to the use of pharmacokinetically derived formulas for dosing carboplatin (39–41) to obtain adequate exposure (AUC) with overall improved therapeutic index. The results of Phase I-II studies with the combination of paclitaxel and carboplatin are intriguing and provocative and hopefully will change the management trends in this disease and create a certain degree of optimism among physicians who treat NSCLC. The recommended doses of carboplatin and paclitaxel in the combination for future studies are as follows: (1) paclitaxel 175 mg/m^2 24-h infusion in combination with carboplatin dose based on a targeted AUC of 7 mg/ml·min using Calvert's formula; (2) paclitaxel 225 mg/m^2 3-h or 1-h infusion in combination

Table 7 Randomized Cooperative Group Studies for Patients with Advanced and Metastatic NSCLC

Study	Schema	Cycle duration
ECOG	Paclitaxel (3 h) 225 mg/m^2/carboplatin AUC = 6 mg/ml·min	3 weeks
	vs.	
	Paclitaxel (24 h) 135 mg/m^2/cisplatin 75 mg/m^2	3 weeks
	vs.	
	Gemcitabine (days 1, 8, 15) 1000 mg/m^2/ cisplatin 100 mg/m^2	4 weeks
	vs.	
	Docetaxel 75 mg/m^2/cisplatin 75 mg/m^2	3 weeks
SWOG	Paclitaxel (3 h) 225 mg/m^2/carboplatin AUC = 6 mg/ml·min vs. navelbine	3 weeks
	25 mg/m^2/wk/cisplatin 100 mg/m^2	4 weeks
CALGB	Paclitaxel (3 h) 225 mg/m^2/carboplatin AUC = 6 mg/ml·min vs. paclitaxel	3 weeks
	(3 h) 225 mg/m^2	3 weeks

with carboplatin dose based on a targeted AUC of 6 or 7 mg/ml·min using Calvert's formula.

This combination regimen of paclitaxel and carboplatin has been incorporated as a part of all ongoing randomized multicenter and cooperative group studies for patients with advanced NSCLC, both in the United States and in Europe (Table 7). A large multicenter randomized study for advanced and metastatic NSCLC comparing the regimen of paclitaxel and carboplatin with cisplatin and etoposide has recently completed accrual (360 patients), and the data are in the process of being analyzed (Table 8). In addition to survival, other endpoints of the study include quality of life alterations and pharmacoeconomic effects on the health care system. These studies, once completed, will hopefully define an effective and optimal regimen for NSCLC.

Table 8 Randomized Comparison of Paclitaxel/Carboplatin Versus Etoposide/Cisplatin in Advanced and Metastatic NSCLC

S	Karnofsky performance status	R	Arm A
T	70–80 vs 90–100	A	Cisplatin 75 mg/m^2 day 1
R		N	Etoposide 1200 mg/m^2
A	Weight loss	D	days 1, 2, 3
T	< 5% vs ≥ 5%	O	(cycles repeated every
I		M	3 weeks)
F	Stage	I	
Y	IIIB vs IV	Z	Arm B
		E	Paclitaxel 225 mg/m^2 (3-h
	Disease measurability		infusion)
	bidimensional vs.		Carboplatin dose AUC =
	unidimensional		6 mg/ml·min
			(cycles repeated every
Study endpoints			3 weeks)
1. Survival			
2. Toxicity			
3. Quality of life			
4. Pharmacoeconomics			

Paclitaxel, in combination with either cisplatin or carboplatin, has become the preferred first-line regimen for advanced and metastatic NSCLC in the United States. These regimens are now being incorporated into combined modality programs with radiation therapy and surgery for the treatment of earlier stages of NSCLC.

REFERENCES

1. Rowinsky EK, Donehower RC. Paclitaxel (Taxol). N Engl J Med 1995; 332:1004–1014.
2. Horwitz SB. Mechanism of action of Taxol. Trends Pharmacol Sci 1992; 13:134–136.
3. Murphy WK, Fossella FV, Winn RJ, et al. Phase II study of taxol in patients with untreated advanced non-small-cell lung cancer. J Natl Cancer Inst 1993; 85:384–388.
4. Chang AY, Kim K, Glick J, et al. Phase II study of taxol, merbarone, and piroxantrone in Stage IV non-small-cell lung cancer: the Eastern Cooperative Oncology Group results. J Natl Cancer Inst 1993; 85:388–394.
5. Gatzemeier U, Heckmayer M, Neuhauss R, et al. Chemotherapy of advanced inoperable non-small cell lung cancer with paclitaxel: a Phase II trial. Semin Oncol 1995; 22(6 suppl 15):24–28.
6. Millward MJ, Bishop JF, Friedlander M, et al. Phase II trial of a 3-hour infusion of paclitaxel in previously untreated patients with advanced non-small-cell lung cancer. J Clin Oncol 1996; 14:142–148.
7. Rowinsky EK, Eisenhauer EA, Chaudhry V, et al. Clinical toxicities encountered with paclitaxel (Taxol). Semin Oncol 1993; 20(4 suppl 3): 1–15.
8. Eisenhauer EA, ten Bokkel Huinink WW, Swenerton KD, et al. European-Canadian randomized trial of paclitaxel in relapsed ovarian cancer: high-dose versus low-dose and long versus short infusion. J Clin Oncol 1994; 12:2654–2666.
9. Hainsworth JD, Thompson DS, Greco FA. Paclitaxel by 1-hour infusion: an active drug in metastatic non-small-cell lung cancer. J Clin Oncol 1995; 13:1609–1614.
10. Hainsworth JD, Raefsky EL, Thomas M, et al. Paclitaxel administered by 1-hr infusion: Phase I/II study comparing two schedules of administration. Proc Am Soc Clin Oncol 1995; 14:A376.

11. Rowinsky EK, Citardi MJ, Noe DA, et al. Sequence-dependent cytotoxic effects due to combinations of cisplatin and the antimicrotubule agents taxol and vincristine. J Cancer Res Clin Oncol 1993; 119: 727–733.

12. Rowinsky EK, Gilbert MR, McGuire WP, et al. Sequences of Taxol and cisplatin: a phase I and pharmacologic study. J Clin Oncol 1991; 9:1692–1703.

13. LeBlanc GA, Sundseth SS, Weber GF, et al. Platinum anticancer drugs modulate p-450 MRNA levels and differentially alter hepatic drug and steroid hormone metabolism in male and female rats. Cancer Res 1992; 52:540–547.

14. Klastersky J, Sculier JP. Cisplatin plus taxol in non-small cell lung cancer: a dose finding trial. Proc Am Assoc Cancer Res 1995; 36:A1423.

15. Pirker R, Krajnik G, Zochbauer S, et al. Paclitaxel-cisplatin in advanced non-small cell lung cancer (NSCLC). Ann Oncol 1995; 6:833–835.

16. Belli L, Le Chevalier T, Gottfried M, et al. Phase I-II trial of paclitaxel (Taxol) and cisplatin in previously untreated advanced non-small cell lung cancer (NSCLC). Proc Am Soc Clin Oncol 1995; 14:A1058.

17. Bonomi PD, Kim K, Chang A, et al. Phase III trial comparing etoposide (E) cisplatin versus Taxol (T) with cisplatin-G-CSF (G) versus cisplatin in advanced non-small cell lung cancer: Eastern Cooperative Oncology Group (ECOG). Proc Am Soc Clin Oncol 1996; 15:A1145.

18. Gelmon KA, Tolcher A, O'Reilly S, et al. Phase I/II trial of biweekly paclitaxel (Taxol) in metastatic breast cancer. Proc Am Soc Clin Oncol 1995; 14:A226.

19. Georgiadis MS, Brown JE, Schuler BS, et al. Phase I study of a four day continuous infusion of paclitaxel followed by cisplatin in patients with advanced lung cancer. Proc Am Soc Clin Oncol 1995; 14:A1072.

20. Lee FH, Cabetta R, Ussekk BF, et al. New platinum complexes in clinical trials. Cancer Treat Rev 1983; 10:43–45.

21. Canetta R, Franks C, Smaldone L, et al. Clinical status of carboplatin. Oncology 1987; 1:61–69.

22. Bonomi PD, Finkelstein DM, Ruckdeschel JC, et al. Combination chemotherapy versus single agents followed by combination chemotherapy in stage IV non-small cell lung cancer: a study of the Eastern Cooperative Oncology Group. J Clin Oncol 1989; 7:1602–1613.

23. Bunn PA Jr. Review of therapeutic trials of carboplatin in lung cancer. Semin Oncol 1989; 16(2 suppl 5):27–33.

24. Klastersky J, Sculier JP, Lacroix H, et al. A randomized study comparing cisplatin or carboplatin with etoposide in patients with advanced

non-small-cell lung cancer: European organization for research and treatment of cancer protocol 07861. J Clin Oncol 1990; 8:1556–1562.

25. Belani CP, Aisner J, Hiponia D, et al. Paclitaxel and carboplatin in metastatic non-small cell lung cancer: preliminary results of a Phase I study. Semin Oncol 1996; 23(5)(suppl 12):19–21.

26. Langer CJ, Leighton JC, Comis RL, et al. Paclitaxel and carboplatin in combination in the treatment of advanced non-small cell lung cancer: a phase II toxicity, response, and survival analysis. J Clin Oncol 1995; 13:1860–1870.

27. Johnson DH, Paul DM, Hande KR, et al. Paclitaxel plus carboplatin in advanced non-small cell lung cancer: a phase II trial. J Clin Oncol 1996; 14:2054–2060.

28. Natale RB. Preliminary results of a phase I/II clinical trial of paclitaxel and carboplatin in non-small cell lung cancer. Semin Oncol 1996; 23(5) (suppl 12):2–6.

29. Rowinsky EK, Flood WA, Sartorius SE, et al. Phase I study of paclitaxel as a 3-hour infusion followed by carboplatin in untreated patients with stage IV non-small cell lung cancer. Semin Oncol 1995; 22(4)(suppl 9):48–54.

30. Schutte W, Bork I, Sucker S. Phase II trial of paclitaxel and carboplatin as firstline treatment in advanced non-small cell lung cancer (NSCLC). Proc Am Soc Clin Oncol 1996; 15:A1208.

31. Bunn PA Jr, Kelly K. A phase I study of carboplatin and paclitaxel in non-small cell lung cancer: a University of Colorado Cancer Center study. Semin Oncol 1995; 22(4 suppl 9):2–6.

32. Giaccone G, Huizing M, Postmus PE, et al. Dose-finding and sequencing study of paclitaxel and carboplatin in non-small cell lung cancer. Semin Oncol 1995; 22:78–82.

33. Hainsworth JD, Thompson DS, Urba WJ, et al. One hour paclitaxel plus carboplatin in advanced non-small cell lung cancer (NSCLC): preliminary results of a multi-institutional phase II study. Proc Am Soc Clin Oncol 1996; 15:A1131.

34. Langer C, Kaplan R, Rosvold E, et al. Paclitaxel (P) by 1 hour (hr) infusion combined with carboplatin (C) in advanced non-small cell lung carcinoma. Proc Am Soc Clin Oncol 1996; 15:A1200.

35. Roa V, Conner A, Mitchell RB. Carboplatin and paclitaxel for chemotherapy-naive patients with advanced non-small cell lung cancer. Proc Am Soc Clin Oncol 1996; 15:A1231.

36. Evans WK, Stewart DJ, Tomiak E, et al. Carboplatin (C) and paclitaxel (P) by one hour infusion for advanced non-small cell lung cancer (NSCLC). Proc Am Soc Clin Oncol 1995; 14:A1156.

37. Kearns CM, Belani CP, Erkmen K, et al. Reduced platelet toxicity with combination carboplatin and paclitaxel; pharmacodynamic modulation of carboplatin associated thrombocytopenia. Proc Am Soc Clin Oncol 1995; 14:A364.
38. Clark JW, Santos-Moore AS, Choy H. Sequencing of Taxol and carboplatinum therapy. Proc Am Assoc Can Res 1995; 36:A1772.
39. Calvert AH, Newell DR, Grumbrell LA, et al. Carboplatin dosage: prospective evaluation of a simple formula based on renal function. J Clin Oncol 1989; 7:1748–1756.
40. Egorin MJ, Van Echo DA, Olman EA, et al. Prospective validation of a pharmacologically based dosing schema for the *cis*-diamminedichloroplatinum (II) analogue diammine cyclobutanedicarboxylatoplatinum. Cancer Res 1985; 45:6502–6506.

13

Paclitaxel/Cisplatin Combination in Inoperable Non-Small-Cell Lung Cancer

European Experience

O. Rixe, L. Belli, and T. Le Chevalier
Institut Gustave Roussy, Villejuif, France

J.-P. Sculier and Jean Klastersky
Jules Bordet Institute, Brussels, Belgium

INTRODUCTION

During the past decade, several cytotoxic drugs have demonstrated interesting activity in the treatment of non-small-cell lung carcinoma (NSCLC); some of them will probably be marketed in the near future both in the United States and in Europe. These new compounds represent an interesting new tool for the treatment of locally advanced or metastatic disease, even in a multimodal approach for operable disease. At the present time, platinum compounds, vinca alkaloids such as vinorelbine, etoposide, 5FU, ifosfamide, and mitomycin C, are the main drugs used in Europe in combination chemotherapy as standard treatments or part of combined modality strategies (1). Taxanes, camptothecin derivatives, and gemcitabine are interesting new drugs that have demonstrated promising activity in lung cancer in first-line chemotherapy for metastatic disease. Since a recent meta-analysis (2) showed a modest but significant improvement in median survival with chemotherapy compared to the best supportive care, new combinations are warranted to substantially modify the poor prognosis of inoperable patients. Paclitaxel has demonstrated a wide spectrum of activity in several human malignancies including ovarian and breast carcinoma, and its efficiency profile should be clarified in NSCLC (3).

Although response rates with multidrug regimens are higher than with single agents, the duration of responses is generally short, even with the most aggressive combinations (4). Cisplatin is one of the most active drugs in NSCLC, with a response rate of approximately 20%, and some literature data suggest a dose-response effect (5). Despite the multiple side effects it can generate, cisplatin is still the standard most effective drug to combine with new compounds for the treatment of advanced NSCLC (2).

Paclitaxel (Taxol; Bristol-Myers Squibb Company, Princeton, NJ), a natural cytotoxic extracted from the bark of *Taxus brevifolia*, has shown promising activity in NSCLC. In 1993, the M.D. Anderson Cancer study has reported the effect of paclitaxel given alone in chemo-naive patients with metastatic NSCLC given at 200 mg/m^2 (6), while the ECOG published a randomized Phase II study using a dose of 250 mg/m^2 given on a 24-h infusion (7). Similar response rates (24% and 21%, respectively) with encouraging 1-year survival lead one to consider paclitaxel as an interesting molecule and open new opportunities for future studies. It is the highest response rate observed with a new agent by the ECOG over the past decade.

In this chapter, we will report the results of the combination of cisplatin and paclitaxel in advanced NSCLC observed in two similar studies, conducted simultaneously at Institut Jules-Bordet (IJB) and Institut Gustave-Roussy (IGR). The rationale for combining cisplatin and paclitaxel includes several biological and clinical reasons: (1) pharmacokinetic interactions and potentiations have been described (8); (2) molecular interactions and preclinical synergisms have been reported (9); (3) each drug used as single agent is effective in NSCLC. This combination has been extensively studied in ovarian cancer (10), becoming in this setting a reference regimen. The two present

Phase I/II studies have evaluated the feasibility and efficacy of pacli-taxel/cisplatin combination in NSCLC with paclitaxel being admin-istered as a 3-h infusion in escalating doses, followed by cisplatin at a dose of 100 or 120 mg/m² as a 1-h infusion every 3 weeks. Their results, which appeared very similar, have been pooled to emphasize our conclusions.

PATIENTS AND METHODS

Population

From March 1993 to May 1994, 49 patients with advanced NSCLC entered these two studies. Patient selection included an age > 18 years with no previous chemotherapy and no histologically proven Stage IIIb or IV NSCLC. The ECOG performance status had to be 2 or less, and at least one measurable lesion was necessary. Adequate hematological (granulocyte count > 1500 109/L, platelet count > 100 × 109/L), hepatic (serum bilirubin level ≤ 1.25 times normal value), renal (serum creatinine level ≤ 1.25 times normal value), and cardiac (no active arrhythmia or congestive heart failure) function were also requested. Patients with brain or leptomeningeal metastases were not allowed to enroll. All patients had to give a written informed consent.

Patients were excluded if they had a past or current history of neoplasm, except for curatively treated basal cell skin carcinoma, documented myocardial affection within the 6 months preceding en-rollment in the study, neurotoxicity World Health Organization grade > 2. Additional exclusions included completion of radiation and/or biological therapy within 4 weeks, mixed non-small-cell and small-cell histology, and previous radiation of more than 30% of marrow-bearing bone.

Treatment

In IGR, paclitaxel was diluted in 500 ml of normal saline and admin-istered as a 3-h infusion via a central catheter, followed 4 h later by cisplatin diluted in 250 ml 3% saline and administered over 1 h with classic hyperhydration. In IJB, paclitaxel was given in 750 ml of normal saline, followed by 250 ml of normal saline (1 h), then cisplatin was administered over 30 min in 250 ml of normal saline followed by a 24-h posthydration (4 L plus osmotic diuresis with mannitol). Premedication consisted of methylprednisolone (10 mg orally 12 and 6 h in IGR) or dexamethasone (20 mg orally 1 and 6 h in IJB) before paclitaxel, promethazine 500 mg or chlorpheniramine 5 mg and cimetidine 300 mg intravenously 30 min before paclitaxel. Antiemetic prophylaxis included dexamethasone, high-dose metoclopramide or ondansetron, and lorazepam or alizapride. Courses were repeated every 3 weeks or after full hematological recovery. Dose levels of paclitaxel were 135, 170, 175, 200, and 225 mg/m^2 with cisplatin 100 mg/m^2, and 200 and 225 mg/m^2 with cisplatin 120 mg/m^2. Grade IV neutropenia lasting > 7 days or any episode of febrile neutropenia prompted a decrease by one dose level. If hematological recovery was not achieved by day 21, the next course was delayed until recovery.

Three patients by level were enrolled. Three additional patients were accrued in case of: neutropenia < 500/mm^3 lasting > 7 days, febrile neutropenia requiring intravenous antibiotics, thrombopenia < 25,000/mm^3, grade 3 mucositis, absence of hematological recovery at day 35, nonhematological toxicity $\geq$ grade 3 (excluding alopecia, vomiting, pain). If two or more patients experienced such a toxicity at a given dose, maximal tolerated dose was considered to be reached and the study was stopped. Chemotherapy was pursued until either disease progression or unacceptable toxicity. In IJB, four additional courses were given in case of complete response; a maximum of 10 courses was planned for partial response.

Patient Evaluation

Toxicity was established through hematological and biochemical tests performed twice a week and clinical examination performed before day 1 of each cycle. Responses were assessed every three cycles by clinical examination and chest x-rays performed every course, and by ultrasound and/or computed tomography scan performed every two courses, according to the target determined at the time of study entry. Toxicity and responses were scored according to the World

Health Organization criteria (11): complete response (complete disappearance of all clinical evidence of the tumor); partial response (decrease of 50% or greater in the sum of the products of the diameters of all measurable lesions); stable disease (decrease of < 50% or increase of < 25% of the sum of all measurable lesions with no new lesions); or progressive disease (25% or greater increase in the sum of the products of perpendicular diameters of measured lesions). Every radiological objective response had to be confirmed with an evaluation by a second independent medical radiologist and had to last at least 4 weeks.

RESULTS

Among 49 patients entered in these studies, there were 33 males and 16 females. Eleven patients had a Stage IIIb disease, and all others had distant metastases. Patient characteristics outlined are presented in Table 1. All patients received at least one cycle. The number of patients by level is reported in Table 2. The maximum number of cycles was 10 in one patient, at the first level.

Toxicity

Major clinical and biological toxicities are listed in Table 3.

First Course

The maximum tolerated dose for the first cycle was not reached. At the third paclitaxel dose level, one patient developed a grade IV neutropenia over 6 days that did not require a specific treatment. At the fourth dose level, one patient had a febrile neutropenia requiring treatment, but this episode was probably related to device rupture with subcutaneous paclitaxel extravasation. The third grade IV neutropenia was noted at the sixth level (200/120 mg/m^2) and did not require hospitalization. During this first course, five patients developed a grade I peripheral neurotoxicity (two patients at the highest dose level).

Table 1 Patient Characteristics

No. of patients	49
Evaluable for response	46
Male/female	33/16
Median age (yr)	59 (25–73)
Median performance status	1 (0–2)
Weight loss > 5%	18
Histology	
Adenocarcinoma	20
Squamous cell carcinoma	19
Large-cell carcinoma	10
AJCC classification	
Stage IIIB	112
Stage IV	38

All Courses

Doses were reduced in one patient each at dose levels 1, 2, and 4 for hematological toxicity (with fever for the two patients at level 1 and 4). Three cycles were delayed for hematological recovery and three cycles for nonhematological toxicity. Neutropenia grade 3 and 4 were observed after 24% and 15% of all cycles, respectively. Nine patients

Table 2 Dosing Information

	Paclitaxel/cisplatin dose level						
	1 135/200 mg/m^2	2 170/100 mg/m^2	3 175/100 mg/m^2	4 200/100 mg/m^2	5 225/100 mg/m^2	6 200/120 mg/m^2	7 225/120 mg/m^2
No. of patients IGR	8	—	6	6	6	—	6
No. of patients IJB	3	3	—	6	—	5	—
Total	11	3	6	12	6	5	6

Table 3 Hematological and Nonhematological Grade III and IV Toxicities (toxicities during all courses: number of patients by dose level)

	Level (no. pts)						
	1 (11)	2 (3)	3 (6)	4 (12)	5 (6)	6 (5)	7 (6)
Neutropenia	4	0	4	4	3	2	3
Thrombopenia	0	0	0	0	0	0	0
Renal toxicity	0	0	0	0	0	0	0
Cardiac toxicity	0	0	0	1	0	2	0

(18%) experienced a grade IV neutropenia. No significant thrombocytopenia was observed, and only one grade II was documented. Three patients became flushed during the first minutes of the paclitaxel infusion. Those hypersensibility reactions were not severe, and neither patient had any reaction during the following courses.

The main cumulative toxicity in this study was the peripheral neurotoxicity. Overall, 28 patients (57%) developed a peripheral neurotoxicity: five were grade I, five were grade II, and 18 were grade III (Table 4). At the highest level, peripheral neurotoxicity occurred in five of the six patients. The median duration of this grade III toxicity was approximately 4 months (range 1 to 11 months). In-

Table 4 Cumulative Grade 3 Neurotoxicity Determined on the 32 Patients Treated in the Gustave-Roussy Study

Dose level	Paclitaxel/ cisplatin	C1	C2	C3	C4	C5	C6	C7	C8	C9	C10
1	135/100	0/6	0/6	0/6	0/5	0/5	0/3	0/3	0/3	2/3	1/1
2	175/100	0/6	0/6	0/5	0/5	0/5	0/3	0/3	1/3	2/2	—
3	200/100	0/6	0/6	0/5	0/5	1/4	1/3	1/2	0/1	—	—
4	225/100	0/6	0/6	0/5	1/4	0/1	0/1	0/1	1/1	—	—
5	225/120	0/6	0/5	0/5	1/5	1/4	2/3	1/1	—	—	—

terestingly, grade III neurotoxicity seemed to occur after the same cumulative dose (whatever the dose level), for a median dose of paclitaxel between 1233 mg/m^2 (level 1) and 1346 mg/m^2 (level 6).

Other toxicities were mild and manageable. Nausea and vomiting grade 1 or 2 appeared in 48% of the courses, and one patient experienced a grade 3 severity (level 1). Alopecia was observed in all patients. Moderate arthralgias and myalgias were observed in 32 cycles, were not dose-dependent, and required treatment in one course at dose level 6. At the first course at level 1, a 44-year-old man died of a bilateral arterial obstruction of lower limbs: a relationship with the treatment could not be excluded. After the first course at dose level 6, one patient experienced transient convulsive seizure, with coma and left hemiplegia after the first cycle. Brain CT scan, MRI, and cerebrospinal fluid were normal. The patient was withdrawn from the study and never recovered completely. One patient at dose level 3 was admitted in intensive care unit for heart arrest, and died a few days later of a fatal hemoptysia. Treatment was stopped in another patient after supraventricular arrhythmia (level 5) in the context of pulmonary thromboembolism after the second cycle. Heart failure related to supraventricular tachycardia was also reported at level 6 in one patient after the third cycle.

Reasons for Withdrawal

Three patients died during the study: two at the level 1 after the first cycle (peritoneal involvement with perforation which was disease-related in one case, and bilateral arterial ischemia in the other case as mentioned previously), one at the level 3 of hemoptysia after the fourth cycle (also previously reported). For the remaining 46 patients, the reasons for withdrawal were toxicity in 22 cases (peripheral neurotoxicity in 19 patients, one central neurotoxicity, and two cases of cardiac and renal toxicities); disease progression in 18 cases; disease progression plus peripheral toxicity in three cases; surgery for resectable thoracic disease in one case; and finally two intercurrent diseases (cerebral infarction and pulmonary thromboembolism).

Efficacy

Of the 46 patients evaluable for response, 19 (41%) had a confirmed partial response. The efficacy of the treatment was superior at the doses of 200 mg/m^2 of paclitaxel and above, objective responses occurring in 48% of cases at these levels. Responses were not related to gender, histological subtype, or disease stage. The median duration of response was 186 days (range 69 to 512 days). Survival was 74% and 24% at 6 months and 1 year, respectively. Median survival was 9 months (95% CI: 7 to 10 months).

DISCUSSION

This study has evaluated the combination of two active drugs in NSCLC and has demonstrated a promising activity. The 41% response rate is high and seems to confirm the synergistic effect of this combination. Used alone, cisplatin has shown response rates in the range of 20% in large studies (12). Paclitaxel has also been reported to give a 24% response rate as first line (13). The existence of a dose-response relationship for paclitaxel in NSCLC has still to be demonstrated (14).

The response rate observed with these two drugs in monotherapy can partially explain the interesting activity of the combination. However, some preclinical data suggest this synergism: Boekelheide et al. (15) demonstrated that cisplatin can interact with cytoskeleton proteins, as tubulin, using a biochemical assay. We recently confirmed this observation (16) on KB epidemoid and A2780 ovarian cell lines: cisplatin as a "Taxol-like" effect and can modify microfilament polymerization in vitro. This inhibition of tubulin depolymerization could partially explain molecular interaction of both drugs on an identical cellular target. In vitro, cisplatin and taxanes have shown synergistic toxicity on several cell lines, including NSCLC (17). Furthermore, molecular mechanisms involved in drug resistance are different for platinum compounds and taxanes: decreased drug accumulation, increased DNA repair, overexpression of detoxifying proteins as glutathion and metallothionein are mainly described in platinum resistance (18), while Pgp (and Pgp-related pumps) and tubulin mutations are involved in taxane resistance (19). This is a way to overcome drug resistance, combining drugs recognized by different patterns of resistance.

Used in such a setting, this combination is one of the most active described in the literature, and compares favorably with other active regimens such as cisplatin/vinorelbine (20) or cisplatin/etoposide (12) in terms of response rates and duration of response. Paclitaxel-cisplatin combination was recently compared to cisplatin-teniposide by the EORTC to assess the real significance of this new combination. A longer follow-up is warranted to analyze this study, which enrolled 251 patients (21). A Phase II study was performed by Krajnik et al. (22) combining paclitaxel at 175 mg/m^2 and cisplatin at 100 mg/m^2. They reported a 35% of objective response rate in 20 patients with a dose-limiting neurotoxicity.

The major toxicity of this combination also was the peripheral neurotoxicity in our study. This is a clear limitation for the use of high doses of paclitaxel and cisplatin and for a prolonged duration of treatment with this combination. This side effect is not surprising as both drugs have a well-established neurotoxicity: in a recent study reported by Chaudry et al. (23), nerve conduction studies have demonstrated the presence of a predominant axonopathy after cisplatin/paclitaxel combination. This toxicity was not directly dose-related and was similar at the different levels of this study. However, the occurrence of this neurological toxicity appears dependent on the cumulative dose of paclitaxel administered. We observed that it was more frequent after a cumulative dose of 1300 mg/m^2. This toxicity seems to be amplified with higher cisplatin doses (120 mg/m^2). As there is no evidence of higher activity for 120 mg/m^2 of cisplatin compared to 100 mg/m^2, and in order to allow a longer duration of treatment, the dose of 100 and 175 mg/m^2 of cisplatin and paclitaxel, respectively, can be suggested.

In conclusion, the combination of paclitaxel and cisplatin is clearly active in advanced NSCLC and compares favorably with the most effective drug combinations. Nevertheless, the peripheral neurotoxicity observed in this cohort of patients, at least at the highest levels, seems a limiting and unavoidable side effect which limits

its use. The combination of paclitaxel with other platinum compounds such as carboplatin or *dach* (diamonocyclohexane) platinum compounds could be an alternative to be clearly evaluated.

REFERENCES

1. Idhe DC, Minna JD. Non-small cell lung cancer. II. Treatment. Curr Probl Cancer 1991; 15:105–154.
2. Non-Small Cell Lung Cancer Collaborative Group. Chemotherapy in non-small cell lung cancer: a metaanalysis using updated data on individual patients from 52 randomised clinical trials. Br Med J 1995; 311: 899–909.
3. Nabholtz JM, Gelmon K, Boutenbal M, et al. Randomized trial of Taxol in metastatic breast cancer: an interim analysis. Proc Am Soc Clin Oncol 1993; 12:61. Abstract.
4. Crino L, Clerici M, Figoli F, et al. Chemotherapy of advanced non-small cell lung cancer: a comparison of three active regimens. A randomized trial of the Italian Oncology Group for Clinical Research (GOIRC). Ann Oncol 1995; 6:347–353.
5. Gralla RJ, Casper ES, Kelsen DP, et al. Cisplatin and vindesine combination chemotherapy for advanced carcinoma of the lung: a randomized trial investigating two dosage schedules. Ann Intern Med 1981; 95: 414–420.
6. Murphy WK, Fossella FV, Winn RJ, et al. Phase II study of Taxol in patients with untreated advanced non-small cell lung cancer. J Natl Cancer Inst 1993; 85:384–387.
7. Chang AY, Kim K, Glick J, et al. Phase II study of Taxol, Merbarone, and piroxantrone in stage IV non-small cell lung cancer: the Eastern Cooperative Oncology Group results. J Natl Cancer Inst 1993; 85:388–394.
8. Rowinsky EK, Gilbert MR, McGuire WP, et al. Sequence of taxol and cisplatin: a phase I and pharmacologic study. J Clin Oncol 1991; 9:1692–1703.
9. Rowinsky EK, Donehower RC. Paclitaxel (Taxol). N Engl J Med 1995; 332:1004–1114.
10. MacGuire WP, Hoskins WJ, Brady MF, et al. Cyclophosphamide and cisplatin compared with paclitaxel and cisplatin in patients with stage III and stage IV ovarian cancer. N Engl J Med 1996; 334:1–6.

11. WHO Handbook for Reporting Results of Cancer Treatment. WHO offset publication 1979; No. 48, Geneva, Switzerland. World Health Organization.

12. Lilenbaum RC, Green MR. Novel chemotherapeutic agents in the treatment of non-small cell lung cancer. J Clin Oncol 1993; 11:1391–1402.

13. Chang AY. Non-small cell lung cancer. In: McGuire WP, Rowinsky EK, eds. Paclitaxel in Cancer Treatment. New York: Marcel Dekker, 1995:273–279.

14. Hainsworth JD, Thompson DS, Greco FA, et al. Paclitaxel by 1-hour infusion: an active drug in metastatic non-small-cell lung cancer. J Clin Oncol 1995; 13:1609–1614.

15. Boekelheide K, Arcila ME, Eveleth J. Cisdiamminedichloroplatinum (II) (cisplatin) alters microtubule assembly dynamics. Toxicol Appl Pharmacol 1992; 116:146–151.

16. Rixe O, Alvarez M, Mickley L, et al. Cisplatin (CP) resistance is multifactorial and includes changes in cytoskeletal distribution and dynamics. Proc Am Assoc Cancer Res 1993; 406. Abstract 2422.

17. Fojo A. Taxanes. In: Pinedo HM, Longo DL, Chabner BA, eds. Cancer Chemotherapy and Biological Response Modifiers Annual 16. Amsterdam: Elsevier, 1996:56–67.

18. Scanlon KJ, Kashani-Sabet M, Miyachi H, et al. Molecular basis of cisplatin resistance in human carcinomas: model systems and patients. Anticancer Res 1989; 9:1301–1312.

19. Horwitz SB, Lothstein L, Manfredi JJ, et al. Taxol: mechanism of action and resistance. Ann NY Acad Sci 1986; 466:733–744.

20. Le Chevalier T, Brisgand D, Douillard J, et al. Randomized study of vinorelbine and cisplatin versus vindesine and cisplatin versus vinorelbine alone in advanced non-small-cell lung cancer: results of a European multicenter trial including 612 patients. J Clin Oncol 1994; 12:360–367.

21. Giaccone G, Splinter T, Postmus P, et al. Paclitaxel-cisplatin versus teniposide-cisplatin in advanced non-small cell lung cancer (NSCLC). Proc Am Soc Clin Oncol 1996; 373. Abstract 1109.

22. Krajnik G, Zöchbauer S, Malayeri R, et al. Paclitaxel/cisplatin in advanced non-small cell lung cancer (NSCLC). Ninth NCI-EORTC symposium on new drugs in cancer therapy, Amsterdam. Ann Oncol 1996; 7(suppl 1):325. Abstract.

23. Chaudry V, Rowinsky EK, Sartorius SE, et al. Peripheral neuropathy from Taxol and cisplatin combination chemotherapy: clinical and electrophysiological studies. Ann Neurol 1994; 35:304–311.

14

Taxanes in Lung Cancer

Combinations of Paclitaxel and Ifosfamide
in Non-Small-Cell Lung Cancer

**Ann M. Mauer, Philip C. Hoffman, Gregory A. Masters,
Harvey M. Golomb, and Everett E. Vokes**
University of Chicago Medical Center, Chicago, Illinois

INTRODUCTION

Current clinical research in non-small-cell lung cancer (NSCLC) involves the evaluation of new antineoplastic agents and the investigation of combination chemotherapy regimens composed of drugs with known single-agent activity and a favorable toxicity spectrum (1). Combination chemotherapy was employed in an attempt to increase the response and survival rates obtained with monotherapies. A goal of current clinical research is to identify new combination regimens that have a more favorable therapeutic index than conventional cisplatin-based regimens.

SINGLE-AGENT PACLITAXEL IN NSCLC

Paclitaxel is one of several new agents identified as active in NSCLC. This drug's novel mechanism of action, the promotion of microtubule

171

assembly and tubulin polymerization, and preclinical activity make it an attractive drug to study. In Phase I studies, the dose-limiting toxicity of paclitaxel was myelosuppression, specifically neutropenia. One study demonstrated that the incidence of severe neutropenia was higher in patients who received a 24-h paclitaxel infusion than for patients who received a 3-h paclitaxel infusion (2). It has been shown that paclitaxel-associated neutropenia is related to the duration of time that plasma paclitaxel concentrations are above a threshold level (3,4).

Several Phase II studies have demonstrated that paclitaxel has significant single-agent activity in stage IV non-small-cell lung cancer with response rates of 21% and 24% (5,6). To date, it has not been determined whether the antitumor activity of paclitaxel varies with the infusion duration for NSCLC. Similarly, it is doubtful that a significant dose response effect exists for paclitaxel in non-small-cell lung cancer. A recent study of paclitaxel at high and low doses in combination with fixed-dose cisplatin offers support that there is no dose response effect for paclitaxel (7). Based on the encouraging responses observed with paclitaxel monotherapy, studies were undertaken to investigate paclitaxel in combination with other active agents in non-small-cell lung cancer.

SINGLE-AGENT IFOSFAMIDE IN NSCLC

Ifosfamide, a cyclophosphamide analog, has demonstrated excellent preclinical activity in a variety of animal tumors including the Lewis lung carcinoma (8). Initial clinical studies of single-agent ifosfamide established its wide range of antitumor activity. In early Phase I studies of ifosfamide, the dose-limiting toxicity was hemorrhagic cystitis. In later studies, where the uroprotectant mesna was administered concurrently, the incidence of urothelial toxicity was greatly diminished without affecting the systemic activity of ifosfamide. When ifosfamide is used in combination with mesna, myelosuppression is the principal dose-limiting toxicity.

Ifosfamide as monotherapy for non-small-cell lung carcinoma has been studied at various dosages and schedules. Several authors have reviewed the efficacy of single-agent ifosfamide in NSCLC (9–12). Several studies employed fractionated dosage schedules of ifosfamide at 1.2 to 2.0 g/m^2 intravenously for 3 to 5 successive days. A schedule of bolus injection ifosfamide at doses of 4.0 to 5.0 g/m^2 for 1 day has also been investigated. In the fractionated dosage and bolus schedules, courses were repeated at 21- to 28-day intervals. For these schedules and dosages of ifosfamide, the response rates ranged from 5% to 35%, with only 2% of patients achieving a complete response. When the studies were considered collectively, the overall response rate was approximately 20% (9,11). At present, the optimal dose and schedule of ifosfamide with mesna for the treatment of NSCLC remain unclear.

COMBINATIONS OF PACLITAXEL AND IFOSFAMIDE

As single agents, paclitaxel and ifosfamide have significant activity in non-small-cell lung cancer. This activity and the overall good tolerability of the agents has led to their use in combination. The paclitaxel/ifosfamide combination has demonstrated activity in other solid tumors, such as ovarian and breast cancer (13–15). To date, two studies investigating the combination of ifosfamide and paclitaxel in advanced non-small-cell lung cancer have been published (16,17).

The first study, conducted at the University of Chicago, evaluated the combination of paclitaxel and ifosfamide in a Phase I dose escalation format (16). As myelosuppression was expected to be the dose-limiting toxicity of the regimen, growth factor support was included in all dose levels. Patients with non-small-cell lung cancer were treated with ifosfamide as a daily bolus infusion on days 1 to 3, and paclitaxel as a 24-h infusion on day 1. Growth factor support with filgrastim (G-CSF) was administered from days 4 through 10 of each 21-day cycle. Paclitaxel doses were escalated from 135 mg/m^2 to 300 mg/m^2 while the ifosfamide dose was fixed at 1.6 g/m^2/day. The dose escalation schema is summarized in Table 1. When the maximum tolerated dose of paclitaxel was identified, the prior dose level (the recommended Phase II dose) was administered in six patients with a paclitaxel infusion duration of only 1 h.

Table 1 Ifosfamide/Paclitaxel with G-CSF Support Dose Escalation Schedule (University of Chicago)

Dose level	Ifosfamide (mg/m^2) IV, day 1, 2, 3	Mesna (mg/m^2) IV with ifosfamide dose, then q4h × 2 doses	Paclitaxel (mg/m^2) IV, day 1
1	1.6	400	130 (24-h infusion)
2	1.6	400	170 (24-h infusion)
3	1.6	400	200 (24-h infusion)
4	1.6	400	250 (24-h infusion)
5	1.6	400	300 (24-h infusion)
6	1.6	400	225 (1-h infusion)

[a]G-CSF support 5 μg/kg SC on days 4–10 (or until ANC > 4000).

Eligibility criteria included histologically or cytologically confirmed diagnosis of NSCLC (stage IIIB and IV) without active brain metastases, and Cancer and Leukemia Group B (CALGB) performance status of 0 to 2. No prior chemotherapy was allowed.

A total of 31 patients participated in the study. The median number of treatment cycles administered was three, with several patients receiving more than six cycles of therapy. The primary toxicity associated with the regimen was neutropenia which was dose-related and evident in all patients who received paclitaxel at the dose level of 300 mg/m². All four patients who received paclitaxel at the dose level of 300 mg/m² had neutropenia. Overall, five patients had neutropenic fever at paclitaxel doses of 170 mg/m², 200 mg/m², and 300 mg/m². Other toxicities were described as mild and of short duration. Toxicity reported included: paroxysmal atrial fibrillation, asymptomatic bradycardia, peripheral neuropathy, neurocortical toxicity, and hyponatremia. Grade 4 hypersensitivity reaction occurred in one patient despite the standard premedication with steroid, H₂-blocker, and antihistamine (see Table 2).

Of the 26 patients evaluable for response, 27% had partial responses. All responses were observed in patients who had received paclitaxel dose levels of at least 250 mg/m². For the regimen, the paclitaxel maximum tolerated dose was defined as 300 mg/m² with

Table 2 Paclitaxel Premedication Schedule

Dexamethasone	20 mg PO 12 h and 6 h prior to paclitaxel infusion
Diphenhydramine	50 mg IV 30 min prior to paclitaxel infusion
Ranitidine	50 mg IV 30 min prior to paclitaxel infusion

the recommended Phase II dose of 250 mg/m^2. The paclitaxel 250 mg/m^2 dose level was expanded to include six additional patients who received the paclitaxel infusion over 1 h without any dose-limiting toxicity. Thus this showed that the regimen could be safely administered in the outpatient setting.

The second paclitaxel/ifosfamide study from the National Cancer Institute of Canada clinical trials group utilized a Phase I dose escalation study to determine the doses of ifosfamide and paclitaxel that could be administered safely without growth factor support (17). Previously untreated patients with advanced non-small-cell lung cancer received paclitaxel as a 3-h infusion and ifosfamide as a 1-h infusion every 3 weeks. The paclitaxel starting dose of 100 mg/m^2 was escalated to a maximum dose of 225 mg/m^2. The ifosfamide starting dose of 3 g/m^2 was fixed until the maximum paclitaxel dose was reached, then the ifosfamide dose was increased to 4 g/m^2. Table 3

Table 3 Ifosfamide/Paclitaxel Dose Escalation Schedule Without G-CSF Support (National Cancer Institute–Canada)

Dose level	Ifosfamide (mg/m^2) IV, day 1	Mesna (mg/m^2) IV with ifosfamide, then q4h × 2 doses	Paclitaxel (mg/m2) IV, 24-h infusion, day 1
1	3	800	100
2	3	800	125
3	3	800	150
4	3	800	175
5	3	800	200
6	3	800	225
7	4	800	225

outlines the dose escalation schema. Eligibility criteria included histologically or cytologically confirmed advanced non-small-cell lung cancer (Stage IIIA, IIIB, or IV) with measurable disease and Eastern Cooperative Oncology Group (ECOG) performance status of 0, 1, or 2. Patients had received no prior chemotherapy and were without central nervous system metastases.

A total of 40 patients participated in the study. Only four of the 164 treatment cycles (2.4%) were delayed due to toxicity. Dose escalation of paclitaxel to 225 mg/m^2 was completed without dose-limiting toxicity; however, the paclitaxel dose was not further escalated to avoid potential neurotoxicity associated with higher doses of paclitaxel. Myelosuppression with dose-related neutropenia of brief duration was observed but not dose-limiting. There was one neutropenic fever and no significant anemia or thrombocytopenia. The nonhematological toxicity described as modest included hematuria, abdominal pain, confusion, paresthesia, and a flu-like syndrome consisting of arthralgia and myalgia. Hypersensitivity reactions, although usually mild, were evident in 37.5%.

Thirty-nine patients were evaluable for response with an overall response rate of 20.5%. All responses were seen in patients treated with paclitaxel doses > 150 mg/m^2. Notably the response rate was 30% for patients treated at paclitaxel doses of 150 mg/m^2 or greater. The recommended doses for Phase II study were paclitaxel 225 mg/m^2 and ifosfamide 4 g/m^2 every 3 weeks.

These studies demonstrate that the combination of paclitaxel and ifosfamide with or without growth factor support can be administered safely in patients with advanced non-small-cell lung cancer. Interestingly, in both studies a dose-related myelosuppression was observed, but neutropenia was dose-limiting only in the study where growth factor was employed. A higher incidence of neutropenic fever was also noted in the study utilizing filgrastim. The reason for this discrepancy is not known, but may be related to the differences in paclitaxel infusion time or ifosfamide scheduling. Overall both regimens were well tolerated, and they can be administered in the outpatient setting.

These investigations also confirm that the combination of paclitaxel and ifosfamide has activity in advanced non-small-cell lung cancer. A Cancer and Leukemia Group B Phase II study of the regimen employing a paclitaxel dose of 250 mg/m^2 on day 1 and a daily ifosfamide dose of 1.6 g/m^2 on days 1 to 3 with filgrastim has recently completed accrual. If significant activity is evident in this Phase II study, the regimen should be compared with the current regimen standard for advanced NSCLC.

The combination of paclitaxel and ifosfamide may also be modified to include other agents with activity in non-small-cell lung cancer. Recently the combination of ifosfamide/vinorelbine has been studied in non-small-cell lung cancer (18). Based on the activity of the paclitaxel/ifosfamide combination and the ifosfamide/vinorelbine combination, further investigation has been undertaken to evaluate the feasibility of a multidrug combination of paclitaxel, ifosfamide, and vinorelbine with growth factor support in non-small-cell lung cancer.

At the present time, the combination of paclitaxel and ifosfamide has not been studied in small-cell lung cancer (SCLC). Paclitaxel and ifosfamide as single agents have each shown significant activity in advanced small-cell lung cancer with response rates of 40% (19,20) and 50% (21), respectively. Thus the combination of paclitaxel and ifosfamide may warrant further investigation in SCLC.

REFERENCES

1. Ginsberg RJ, Vokes EE, Raben A. Cancer of the lung. In: DeVita VT, Hellman S, Rosenberg SA, eds. Cancer: Principles & Practice of Oncology. 5th ed. Philadelphia: Lippincott, 1997:858–911.
2. Eisenhauer EA, ten Bokkel Huinink WW, Swenerton KD, et al. European-Canadian randomized trial of paclitaxel in relapsed ovarian cancer: high-dose versus low-dose and long versus short infusion. J Clin Oncol 1994; 12:2654–2666.
3. Gianni L, Kearns CM, Giani A, et al. Nonlinear pharmacokinetics and metabolism of paclitaxel and its pharmacokinetic/pharmacodynamic relationships in humans. J Clin Oncol 1995; 13:180–190.
4. Huizing MT, Keung AC, Rosing H, et al. Pharmacokinetics of paclitaxel and metabolites in a randomized comparative study in platinum-treated ovarian cancer patients. J Clin Oncol 1993; 11:2127–2135.

5. Murphy WK, Fossella FV, Winn RJ, et al. Phase II study of taxol in patients with untreated advanced non-small cell lung cancer. J Natl Cancer Inst 1993; 85:384–388.

6. Chang AY, Kim Y, Glick J, et al. Phase II study of taxol, merbarone, and piroxantrone in stage IV non-small cell lung cancer: the Eastern Cooperative Oncology Group results. J Natl Cancer Inst 1993; 85:388–394.

7. Bonomi P, Kim K, Chang A, et al. Phase III trial comparing etoposide cisplatin versus taxol with cisplatin-G-CSF versus taxol cisplatin in advanced non-small cell lung cancer. An Eastern Cooperative Oncology Group study. Proc Am Soc Clin Oncol 1996; 15:382. Abstract 1145.

8. Golden A. Ifosfamide in experimental tumor systems. Semin Oncol 1982; 9(suppl 1):14–23.

9. Ettinger DS. Ifosfamide in the treatment of non-small cell lung cancer. Semin Oncol 1989; 16(suppl 3):31–38.

10. Drings P. European experience with ifosfamide in non-small cell lung cancer. Semin Oncol 1989; 16(suppl 3):22–30.

11. Johnson DH. Overview of ifosfamide in small cell and non-small cell lung cancer. Semin Oncol 1990; 17(suppl 4):24–30.

12. Eberhardt W, Niederle N. Ifosfamide in non-small cell lung cancer: a review. Semin Oncol 1992; 19(suppl 1):40–48.

13. Murad AM, Tinoco LA, Schwartsmann WC. Phase II trial of the use of taxol and ifosfamide in heavily pre-treated patients with metastatic breast cancer. Proc Am Soc Clin Oncol 1996; 15:97. Abstract 52.

14. Pucci F, Bella M, Salvagni S, et al. Paclitaxel and ifosfamide in heavily pretreated patients with advanced ovarian cancer. A pilot phase II study. Proc Am Soc Clin Oncol 1996; 15:301. Abstract 838.

15. Klaassen U, Harstrick A, Stahl M, et al. Paclitaxel and ifosfamide in pretreated patients with advanced ovarian carcinoma—results of a phase I/II study. Proc Am Soc Clin Oncol 1996; 15:295. Abstract 813.

16. Hoffman PC, Masters GA, Drinkard LC, et al. Ifosfamide plus paclitaxel in advanced non-small cell lung cancer: a phase I study. Ann Oncol 1996; 7:314–316.

17. Shepard FA, Latreille J, Crump M, et al. Phase I study of paclitaxel (Taxol®) and ifosfamide in previously untreated patients with advanced non-small-cell lung cancer. Ann Oncol 1996; 7:311–313.

18. Masters DA, Hoffman PS, Hsieh A, et al. Phase I study of vinorelbine and ifosfamide in advanced non-small-cell lung cancer. J Clin Oncol 1997; 15:884–892.

19. Ettinger DS, Finkelstein DM, Sarma R, Johnson DH. Phase II study of Taxol in patients with extensive-stage small cell lung cancer: an Eastern Cooperative Oncology Group study. J Clin Oncol 1995; 13: 1430–1435.

20. Jett JR, Kirschling RJ, Jung SH, Marks RS. A phase II study of paclitaxel and granulocyte colony-stimulating factor in previously untreated patients with extensive-stage small cell lung cancer: a study of the North Central Cancer Treatment Group. Semin Oncol 1995; 22(suppl 6): 75–77.

21. Ettinger DS. The place of ifosfamide in chemotherapy of small cell lung cancer: the Eastern Cooperative Oncology Group experience and a selected literature update. Semin Oncol 1995; 22(suppl 2):23–27.

15

Taxanes and Radiation Therapy in Solid Tumors

Hak Choy
Vanderbilt University Medical Center, Nashville, Tennessee

W. Akerley
Rhode Island Hospital, Providence, Rhode Island

H. Safran
Miriam Hospital, Providence, Rhode Island

INTRODUCTION

Combination therapy with taxanes and radiation has only recently been introduced to clinical trials of lung cancer and other malignancies. Extensive trial work from the pretaxane era to evaluate the significance of in vitro synergy between chemotherapy and radiation favors overall a beneficial effect from combined therapy in the treatment of solid tumors. Laboratory studies suggest that the taxanes as a group may be more effective as potentiators of radiation than previous agents, but their interactions are complex and our understanding continues to evolve. Clinical trials with taxanes and radiation have been initiated to evaluate their effectiveness and role in the treatment of solid tumors.

RADIATION AND CHEMOTHERAPY IN
PRIMARY TREATMENT OF LUNG CANCER

Various agents, but especially cisplatin in the pretaxane era, have been used either sequentially or concurrently in clinical trials of combined chemoradiotherapy for advanced non-small-cell lung cancer (NSCLC). CALBG 8433 was the first major randomized clinical trial to demonstrate the significant survival advantage for the combination of sequential chemotherapy and radiation for patients with inoperable stage III NSCLC (1). The treatment consisted of 6000 cGy in 200 cGy fractions with or without two cycles of prior cisplatin and weekly vinblastine for 5 weeks. Response rates were 56% for patients receiving combination therapy and 43% for patients receiving radiation alone with median survivals of 13.7 and 9.6 months ($p = .0066$). Reanalysis of this trial at 7 years showed these findings to persist with 5-year survivals of 17% versus 6%, respectively (2). The trial has also been confirmed independently in an intergroup trial by the RTOG/ECOG with similar findings of improved 1 year and median survivals of 60% and 13.8 months versus 46% and 11.4 months for combined therapy over radiation alone, respectively (3). In another randomized study demonstrating improvement in 3-year survival for sequential chemoradiotherapy over radiation alone (4), a decreased frequency of distant relapses was noted (5).

Concomitant chemoradiotherapy offers an alternative strategy for combined therapy. Its potential advantages over sequential therapy are the immediate treatment of both local and distant sites of disease simultaneously and the opportunity for synergy between the modalities to enhance local control (6). These must be balanced against the potential for enhancement of toxicity to normal tissues. The principle of synergy between concomitant radiation and chemotherapy is well described in vitro (7), but more difficult to prove in clinical practice. In a three-arm, randomized trial in Stage III inoperable NSCLC by the EORTC, patients were treated with radiation alone (split course: 55 Gy in 20 fractions with a 3- to 4-week mid-course break), identical radiation plus cisplatin at 30 mg/m²/week during radiation, or radiation plus cisplatin at 6 mg/m²/day with identical total doses of cisplatin (8). While overall response rates were similar for all three arms, there was an improvement in overall survival for radiation plus cisplatin over radiation alone ($p = .04$) and particularly for radiation plus daily cisplatin compared with radiation only ($p < .009$). Analyses of patterns of failure showed improvement was confined to regional control. A recent meta-analysis (9) evaluating multiple clinical trials from the pretaxane era confirms the overall beneficial effect of combined therapy over radiation alone. These benefits in survival are greatest when cisplatin is included in the chemotherapy regimen and are likely influenced by study design and pretreatment characteristics (10).

THE TAXANES

The taxanes are a new class of plant-derived antineoplastic compounds which share a unique mechanism of cytotoxic action and significant demonstrable efficacy in a wide variety of malignancies (11–20). Paclitaxel and docetaxel are the first members of this class to be used in clinical practice. They act by promoting assembly of microtubules and rendering the microtubules resistant to depolymerization (21–23). Microtubules function not only in mitotic spindle formation, but also in many vital interphase functions of the cell, including maintenance of shape, motility, anchorage, mediation of signals between surface receptors and the nucleus, and intracellular transport (24,25). Consequently, interference of these actions may cause irreversible damage initiating apoptosis and/or resulting in arrest of cells in the G2M phases of the cell cycle, the phases with particular sensitivity to radiation (26). Both actions have the potential to contribute to enhanced radiation effect. Although limited experience in combined modality therapy exists, these attributes provide strong support for the clinical application of taxanes with radiation.

MECHANISMS OF RADIATION-ENHANCING EFFECTS OF PACLITAXEL

Significant efforts have been focused on the ability of taxanes to potentiate the effects of radiation. While support exists for several potential mechanisms of interaction in vitro, cell synchronization appears to be the dominant factor (27–32). Paclitaxel, the prototype taxane, is extremely effective in causing arrest of tumor cells in the G2/M phase of the cell cycle. After only brief and low-level exposure to paclitaxel at concentrations of 30 nm for 1 h, arrest of proliferating cells in G2M can be noted starting as early as 4 h and approach a maximum of 70% at 24 h. These concentrations are routinely exceeded by 100 in the plasma and are achievable within the tumor in clinical practice (33). The fraction of arrested cells increases as a function of both concentration and duration of exposure (34).

Following treatment with paclitaxel and consequent synchronization of tumor cells, enhanced sensitivity to radiation can be demonstrated in many cell lines. In the study by Choy et al., HL-60 cells after 1 h exposure at 30 nM, the sensitizer enhancement ratio (SER) was increased to 1.5 (50% greater cell kill at equal doses of radiation after correcting for direct effects of paclitaxel) (27).

Summary of Other Experiments (duration sentence and concentration sentence, differences in cell lines)

With greater duration of exposure for 24 h at 10 nM Taxol, the SER was increased to 1.8 and at 50 nM, the ratio approaches 2.0 in PC-3 cells.

Enhancement of radiation response by taxanes may also occur through additional mechanisms independent of cell cycle synchronization. Recently, Lieberman et al. (29) have shown that the G2M cell cycle block alone may not be sufficient for Taxol-induced radiation sensitization in other human tumor cells. A good correlation between G2M arrest and degree of radiation sensitization, however, was obtained with the other cell lines tested in in vitro studies (26,33).

Several groups have shown that mechanisms other than the paclitaxel-induced cell cycle perturbation must exist, at least in the in vivo setting, by which paclitaxel potentiates cellular radio response. Milas et al. addressed a possibility that paclitaxel makes tumor cells more susceptible to radiation-induced apoptosis (36). There is increasing evidence that various anticancer agents, including radiation (35,36) and chemotherapeutic drugs (37,38), induce apoptosis in tumors and that paclitaxel is capable of inducing a strong apoptotic response in murine tumors, including the MCA-4 tumors (39). Pacli-taxel-induced apoptosis developed mainly from mitotically arrested cells. Because development of apoptosis after paclitaxel treatment depended on mitotic arrest, the pattern of development of apoptosis was similar to the kinetics of mitotic arrest, the difference being that the development of apoptosis lags several hours behind that of mi-totic arrest. The apoptotic response induced by paclitaxel persists for about 2 days. In contrast to paclitaxel, radiation-induced apoptosis in MCA-4 tumors increased rapidly so that the peak in apoptotic response occurred 4 h after irradiation. Radiation-induced apoptosis rapidly declined, approaching the background level by 12 h after ir-radiation. The efficacy of radiation in inducing apoptosis in tumors treated with paclitaxel depended on the time when radiation was delivered after paclitaxel administration or whether cells were in mi-tosis at the time of irradiation. Radiation delivered 1 h after pacli-taxel, when only a low percentage of cells were in mitosis, was not more effective in inducing apoptosis than in tumors not treated with paclitaxel. However, when radiation was given 9 or 24 h after pacli-taxel, when many cells were in mitosis, there was a significant in-crease in radiation-induced apoptosis.

An alternative explanation is that treatment with paclitaxel re-sults in reoxygenation of hypoxic tumor cells, a reoxygenation that increases with time. About one-third of total tumor cell population becomes mitotically arrested within 9 h after paclitaxel administration, and the majority of these cells die by apoptosis or other modes of cell death (40). The dead cells are rapidly removed from the tumor so that at 24 h after paclitaxel, the MCA-4 tumor was histologically depopu-lated. It is logical to anticipate that this removal of dead cells should result in tumor reoxygenation, which makes tumor cells two or three times more sensitive to radiation (40). Since about 30% of cells in 8-mm MCA-4 tumors are hypoxic (41) in untreated air-breathing mice, their reoxygenation would considerably increase tumor radio response. The in vivo study by Milas et al. showed that paclitaxel reduced radiobiological hypoxia in tumors, a major cause of tumor cell resistance to radiation, and that the induced reoxygenation in-creased as the time between administration of paclitaxel and tumor irradiation increased within the observation period of 3 days (42).

In summary, the taxanes interact with radiation at many levels. Cell cycle synchronization through mitotic arrest has been consistently shown to play a major role in radiation enhancement, but increased apoptosis and tumor reoxygenation may constitute additional mechanisms. Clearly, the interaction is multifactorial interaction, and the dominant mechanism may be affected by specifics of the setting including drug exposure and concentration, tumor type, and radiation dosimetry.

CLINICAL EXPERIENCE WITH PACLITAXEL AND RADIATION

Phase I Trials

We have recently performed and completed three Phase I trials of paclitaxel with concurrent radiation for three separate organ sites. In each trial the paclitaxel was administered weekly over 3 h with standard premedication for 6 weeks with daily radiation. The weekly schedule of paclitaxel was chosen to increase the duration and frequency of temporal overlap between the taxane and radiation for maximal potential interaction. The purpose of each was to determine the maximum tolerated dose and dose-limiting toxicities. In each trial, there was a similar and distinct toxicity profile of minimal myelosuppression and neuropathy.

In the Phase I trial of weekly paclitaxel and radiation for Stage III NSCLC, paclitaxel was initiated at 10 mg/m^2/week with dose escalation of 10 mg/m^2 in each successive group of three new patients as tolerated (43). Dose-limiting toxicity was defined as grade 3 or 4 nonhematological toxicity excluding nausea and vomiting or grade 4 hematological toxicity according to CALGB expanded common toxicity criteria. Thoracic radiation was administered for 6 weeks with original and boost volumes irradiated sequentially. The dose to the original volume was 40 Gy in 20 fractions of 200 cGy, the boost volume dose was 20 Gy in 10 fractions. Eligible patients had inoperable stage III or stage IV disease limited to previously treated brain metastases.

Twenty-seven patients were accrued to seven dose levels ranging from 10 to 70 mg/m^2/week. Esophagitis was the principal dose-limiting toxicity of the paclitaxel-radiation combination in lung cancer patients (Table 1). Grade 4 esophagitis with hospitalizations for IV hydration and analgesic administration occurred in two of three patients at 70 mg/m²/week dose level. In the expanded 60 mg/m² level, one of seven patients developed grade 3 esophagitis and three developed grade 2 esophagitis. Despite an aggregate paclitaxel dose of 210 mg/m² per 21 days, only one patient developed grade 3 neutropenia (Table 2) without fever, and there were no episodes of complete alopecia or neuropathy. There was no apparent added pulmonary toxicity from concurrent therapy. Four of 23 evaluable patients had a complete response (17%), and 13 achieved a partial response (56%), for an overall objective response rate of 73% (95% confidence interval 65% to 83%). Paclitaxel at 60 mg/m²/week was recommended as the Phase II dose level for further evaluation.

In a second Phase I trial, increasing doses of paclitaxel and concurrent cranial irradiation (60 Gy) were administered to sequential cohorts of adults with primary brain tumors (44). Sixty patients were treated with doses of paclitaxel ranging from 20 to 275 mg/m²/week × 6. Fifty-six completed the prescribed course of therapy. The dose-limiting toxicity in this study was peripheral neuropathy (Table 3) which occurred to some degree in 25% (14 of 56) of patients. The

Table 1 Nonhematological Toxicity in Phase I Study of Weekly Paclitaxel and RT for NSCLC

Dose (mg/m²)	No. patients	Esophagitis				Dermatitis grade				Myalgias			
		1	2	3	4	1	2	3	4	0	1	2	3
10	3	1	2	0	0	2	1	0	0	2	1	0	0
20	3	2	1	0	0	3	0	0	0	2	1	0	0
30	3	3	0	0	0	3	0	0	0	2	1	0	0
40	2	3	0	0	0	3	0	0	0	3	0	0	0
50	3	2	1	0	0	1	1	1	0	2	1	0	0
60	7	3	3	1	0	5	2	0	0	5	2	0	0
70	3	0	1	0	2	1	1	1	0	2	1	0	0

Source: Ref. 43.

Table 2 Hematological Toxicity (median nadirs) in Phase I Study of Weekly Paclitaxel and RT for NSCLC

Dose (mg/m^2)	No. patients	Hbg (range) (g/dL)	WBC (range) ($\times 10^3$/mL)	PLT (range) ($\times 10^3$/mL)
10	3	11.4 (10.7–14.4)	3.6 (3.2–5.7)	313 (265–352)
20	3	13.8 (10.8–15.4)	5.6 (4.6–8.8)	179 (133–301)
30	3	12 (11–13.4)	5.4 (4.7–6.5)	348 (170–374)
40	2	10.6 (9.9–11.3)	3.3 (2.7–3.0)	215 (140–291)
50	3	9.4 (8.8–14)	4.1 (1.8–5.1)	161 (48–198)
60	7	10.7 (8.9–12.7)	3.3 (2.1–6.3)	174 (144–347)
70	3	11.9 (10.8–12.8)	2.6 (1.2–5.5)	150 (144–301)

Source: Ref. 43.

frequency and severity of neuropathy were related to dose, and all patients with grade 3 neuropathy received the 275 mg/m^2 dose level. Neuropathic symptoms continued to progress for 1 to 3 weeks after therapy and subsequently improved in all patients. Only four patients continued to report symptoms of symmetrical mild numbness

Table 3 Nonhematological Toxicity in Phase I Study of Weekly Paclitaxel and RT for Primary Brain Tumors

Dose level (mg/m^2/course)	No. patients	Cutaneous toxicity grade				Sensory neuropathy grade			Pruritus grade		
		1	2	3	4	1	2	3	1	2	3
20–150	39	0	0	0	0	0	0	0	0	0	0
175	5	0	0	0	1[a]	1	2	0	0	0	0
200	4	0	0	0	0	0	0	0	0	0	0
225	3	1	1	1	0	1	2	0	0	0	1
250	6	1	1	0	0	2	3	0	0	1	1
275	3	0	1	1	0	0	1	2	0	0	1
Total	60	2	3	2	1	4	8	2	0	1	3

Source: Ref. 44.
[a]1 = mild, 2 = moderate, 3 = severe (no formal CALGB criteria available).

Table 4 Hematological Toxicity in Phase I Study of Weekly Paclitaxel and RT for Primary Brain Tumors

Dose level (mg/m²/course)	No. patients	ANC grade 1	2	3	Thrombocytopenia grade 1,2	3,4	Anemia grade 1	2	3,4
20	3	0	0	0	0	0	1	0	0
30	3	0	0	0	0	0	0	0	0
40	3	0	1	0	0	0	0	1	0
50	3	0	1	0	0	0	1	0	0
60	3	0	0	0	0	0	0	2[a]	0
70	3	1	0	0	0	0	1	1	0
80	3	0	0	0	0	0	1	0	0
90	2	0	0	0	0	0	1	0	0
100	3	0	0	0	0	0	1	0	0
110	3	0	0	0	0	0	0	0	0
135	3	0	0	0	1	0	0	0	0
150	3	0	0	0	1	0	2	0	0
175	5	1	0	1[b]	2	0	1	1	0
200	4	1	0	0	1	0	4	0	0
225	3	2	0	0	0	0	1	0	0
250	6	0	1	0	0	0	4	0	0
275	3	0	1	0	1	0	2	0	0
Total	56	5	4	1	6	0	20	5	0

Source: Ref. 44.
[a]Secondary to gastrointestinal bleeding in one patient.
[b]Patient died of aspiration pneumonia following a stroke.

of the toes. Decreased vibratory sensation has persisted in all patients with grade 2 or 3 neuropathy.

Hematological toxicity was unexpectedly mild and never required a dose reduction or treatment delay (Table 4). The nadir of the absolute neutrophil count occurred most frequently during the third week of treatment, and only four patients developed grade 2 neutropenia. No patient experienced greater than grade 2 anemia or grade 1 thrombocytopenia. Other toxicities included a 2- to 4-week occurrence of a self-limited, diffuse, painless erythema of the skin which developed in eight patients (15%) and progressed to ulceration in only one (Table 3).

Plasma pharmacokinetic studies were performed on 10 patients and were found to closely resemble those previously described for women with breast or ovarian cancer receiving 3-h infusions of paclitaxel. In terms of AUC and duration of paclitaxel concentration above 0.05 mMol/L. However, these values did not correlate with expected percent reductions in absolute neutrophil counts from previous studies. The reductions expected from just the first week's dose of paclitaxel are much greater than those actually observed after all six doses administered in this study. The explanation for this deviation in pharmacodynamics remains obscure. Although most patients in this trial also received daily corticosteroids and anticonvulsants which might theoretically induce the P-450 enzyme systems and affect paclitaxel clearance, our data did not support altered pharmacokinetics as the major explanation for the unexpectedly mild neutropenia observed. Other trials have demonstrated conflicting results.

These Phase I studies show that treatment with taxane and concurrent radiation is feasible in a wide variety of malignancies. In addition, it would appear that paclitaxel delivered on a 7-day schedule is less toxic than the conventional 21-day schedule. The dose-limiting toxicities from these trials occurred within the radiation field at a rate greater than expected and provide evidence for some degree of interaction between the modalities which warrant Phase II evaluation.

Phase II Study of Weekly Taxol and RT for NSCLC

Previously untreated patients with histologically documented inoperable Stage IIIA or Stage IIIB NSCLC were entered in this study (45). Patients with direct vertebral body invasion or a malignant or exudative pleural effusion were not eligible. All patients had measurable or assessable disease. Paclitaxel 60 mg/m^2 was administered weekly as a 3-h IV infusion in the outpatient setting for 6 weeks. Paclitaxel was usually given at the beginning of the week, prior to the first weekly dose of radiation treatment. Radiation was delivered as 200 cGy fractions 5 days weekly for 6 weeks. The original and boost volumes were irradiated sequentially. Treatment volume and dose were same as Phase I study.

Thirty-three patients entered this study. The age range was 40 to 80 years and the median age was 68. There were 19 males and 14 females. Twelve patients had Stage IIIA disease, and 21 had Stage IIIB. The most common histological type was squamous carcinoma (55%). Most patients had a CALGB performance status of 1.

Of the 33 patients enrolled, four were inevaluable. One patient was removed from the study after the discovery of subcutaneous metastatic disease during the first week of treatment. Two patients withdrew from the study during the second week of treatment due to disease progression in one patient and the other patient's refusal to receive any additional chemotherapy. One patient developed a hypersensitivity reaction to her first dose of paclitaxel and was not rechallenged. The remaining 29 patients form the basis of this report.

Twenty-seven of 29 patients received all six paclitaxel treatments. Two patients received only five treatments due to esophagitis. Thus a total of 172 cycles of weekly paclitaxel were administered for the 29 evaluable patients, or 99% of the planned paclitaxel doses. Twenty-seven of 29 patients received the planned 60 Gy radiation. Radiation dosage was reduced to 48 and 50 Gy in two patients due to esophagitis.

The complete response rate was 7% (2/29) and the partial response rate was 79% (23/29) for an overall response rate of 86% (95% confidence interval, 68% to 95%). Three patients had stable disease (10%). One patient had local tumor progression on chest CT scan at completion of treatment.

All subgroups responded favorably, and no statistically significant differences were noted with regard to performance status, histology, or stage. The response rate was 100% for women and 78% for men. The most frequent histological subtype in this trial was squamous cell carcinoma. Fourteen of 17 patients with squamous cell carcinomas responded (82%). All seven patients with adenocarcinoma had at least partial responses (100%). Patients with stage IIIB disease responded equally well as patients with stage IIIA disease.

Esophagitis was the most significant toxicity noted in this study. Six patients (20%) had grade 3 esophagitis (requiring narcotics in order to eat solids). Five patients (17%) had grade 4 esophagitis, defined as the requirement for parenteral or enteral support or the need for hospitalization for intravenous hydration. Only one patient required a jejunostomy tube for enteral nutrition to complete therapy, and no patient required total parenteral nutrition (TPN). Esophagitis generally began in the final 2 weeks of treatment and resolved within 2 weeks of completing treatment in all patients. Two patients had grade 2 peripheral neuropathy, characterized by numbness and hypesthesia of the hands and feet, which resolved within a few weeks of completing treatment. Two patients had significant pulmonary toxicity. These patients had pneumonitis with shortness of breath, hypoxia, and interstitial infiltrates. The pneumonitis improved rapidly with corticosteroids. The only significant hematological toxicity was grade 3 neutropenia in two patients. One patient had a fever that persisted for 4 weeks during treatment as an outpatient without an identified source of infection. One patient had a grade 3 supraventricular tachycardia with a near syncopal episode. No other cardiac toxicity was observed. One patient had a grade 3 hypersensitivity reaction during her first cycle of paclitaxel with hypotension and rash and was not retreated. No patient had grade 3 or 4 nausea, vomiting, or complete alopecia.

The overall median survival time has not yet been reached in this study. At a median follow-up of 12 months, the overall survival rate was 73% (95% CI: 66% to 96%). This Phase II study of concurrent paclitaxel/RT for patients with Stage III NSCLC demonstrated an 86% overall response rate. Responses were noted in all subgroups. There was no statistically significant difference in response rates according to gender, histology, or stage.

Although mean follow-up in this study is just 12 months, our overall response rate is promising and comparable to the most active chemoradiation combinations recently reported, including the 38% response rate observed with radiation alone in the control arm of the Hoosier Oncology Group study (46) or the 45% response rate reported by Perez for locally advanced NSCLC (38). Our current response rate is also much greater than the 20 to 25% response rate anticipated from paclitaxel as a single agent (16,17). Thus, the substantial response rate seen with concurrent paclitaxel/RT appears to justify the clinical use of concurrent RT/paclitaxel and is suggestive, though not conclusive, for a radiation enhancement effect.

ROLE OF p53 IN CONCURRENT PACLITAXEL AND RADIATION THERAPY

Apoptosis, or programmed cell death, is the major mechanism by which ionizing radiation and most chemotherapeutic agents cause tumor cell death (47). Wild-type p53 function is required in vitro to induce apoptosis by wide variety of chemotherapeutic agents and radiation (48,49). Mutations in the p53 gene typically result in an abnormal protein that usually has a longer life than the wild-type protein (49). Mutant p53 protein may also inactivate wild-type protein (50–52). These features make p53 a potentially critical determinant of therapeutic response. Mutations in p53 are associated with resistance to chemotherapy in patients with NSCLC and other malignancies (53–58).

We have conducted p53 mutation analysis from tumor samples of patients who participated in the paclitaxel and radiation studies (59). All mutations were confirmed in an independent PCR/SSCP assay. We observed nearly identical response rates (complete plus partial responses) to paclitaxel/RT in patients with and without p53 mutations. A 75% response rate (9 of 12; 95% CI 43 to 95%) was observed for tumors with p53 mutations, as compared with an 83% response rate for tumors without evidence of p53 mutations (15 of 18; 95% CI, 59% to 96%; $p = .7$).

p53 Gene mutations do not predict response to paclitaxel/RT in NSCLC. This finding is in marked contrast to the dependence of other chemotherapeutic agents and radiotherapy on wild-type p53 and suggests a unique mechanism of action for this therapy. These results provide clinical support for in vitro observations that paclitaxel can bypass mutant p53 and lead to tumor cell death by alternate pathway(s). These findings further suggest that paclitaxel/RT may be an active regimen for other neoplasms with frequent p53 gene mutations. Studies are ongoing to evaluate p53 mutations for patients receiving paclitaxel/RT with locally advanced pancreatic and gastric tumors (60).

CONCLUSION

Paclitaxel/RT was safely administered on an outpatient basis. The toxicity was acceptable and compared favorably with other regimens currently used. Based on this response and toxicity profile, we believe concurrent RT/paclitaxel offers significant clinical utility for control of both local and distant spread.

Several new studies using a weekly schedule of paclitaxel administration are under way. Phase II trials of weekly paclitaxel and carboplatin and RT are also under way in multiple tumor sites.

We are extending our investigation of concurrent weekly paclitaxel and radiation therapy to the neoadjuvant setting for patients with potentially resectable minimal N2 disease. We feel that early institution of effective local and systemic therapy will eventually translate into improvements in survival.

REFERENCES

1. Dillman RO, Seagren SL, Propert K, et al. A randomized trial of induction chemotherapy plus high-dose radiation versus radiation alone in stage III non-small cell lung cancer. N Engl J Med 1990; 323:940–945.
2. Dillman RO, Herdon J, Seagren S, et al. Improve survival in Stage III non-small cell lung cancer: CALBG8433. J Natl Cancer Inst 1996; 88: 1210–1215.
3. Sause WT, Scott C, Taylor S, et al. Radiation Therapy Oncology Group (RTOG) 88-08 and Eastern Cooperative Oncology Group (ECOG) 4588: preliminary results of a Phase III trial in regionally advanced, unresectable non-small-cell lung cancer. J Natl Cancer Inst 1995; 87:198–205.
4. Le Chevalier T, Arriagada R, Quoix E, et al. Radiotherapy alone versus combined chemotherapy and radiotherapy in nonresectable non-small-cell lung cancer. First analysis of a randomized trial in 353 patients. J Natl Cancer Inst 1991; 83:417–423.
5. Le Chevalier T, Arriagada R, Lacombe-Terrier M-J, et al. Significant effect of adjuvant chemotherapy on survival in locally advanced non-small-cell lung carcinoma. J Natl Cancer Inst 1992; 84:58.
6. Vokes E, Weichselbaum R. Concomitant chemoradiotherapy: rationale and clinical experience in patients with solid tumors. J Clin Oncol 1990; 8:911–934.

7. Skov K, MacPhail S. Interaction of platinum drugs with clinically rere-valent X-ray doses in mammalian cells: a comparison of cisplatin, car-boplatin, iproplatin, and tetraplatin. Int J Radiat Oncol Biol Phys 1991; 20:221–225.

8. Schaake-Koning C, van den Bogaert W, Dalesio O, et al. Effects of concomitant cisplatin and radiotherapy on inoperable non-small cell lung cancer. N Engl J Med 1992; 326(8):524–530.

9. Marino P, Preatoni A, Cantoni A. Randomized trials of radiotherapy alone versus combined chemotherapy and radiotherapy in stages IIIa and IIIb nonsmall cell lung cancer. A meta-analysis. Cancer 1995; 76(4):593–601.

10. Paesmans M, Sculier JP, Libert P, et al. Prognostic factors for survival in advanced non-small-cell lung cancer: univariate and multivariate analyses including recursive partitioning and amalgamation algorithms in 1,052 patients. J Clin Oncol 1995; 13:1221–1230.

11. McGuire WP, Rowinsky EK, Rosenshein NB, et al. Taxol. Int Med 1989; 111:273.

12. Holmes F, Walters R, Theriault R, et al. Phase II trial of Taxol, an active drug in metastatic breast cancer. J Natl Cancer Inst 1991; 83: 1797.

13. Reichman B, Seidman A, Crown J, et al. Paclitaxel and recombinant human granulocyte-colony-stimulating factor as initial chemotherapy for metastatic breast cancer. J Clin Oncol 1993; 11:1943.

14. Seidman A, Crown J, Reichman B, et al. Lack of cross-resistance of Taxol (T) with anthracycline (A) in the treatment of metastatic breast cancer (MBC). Proc Am Soc Clin Oncol 1993; 12:63. Abstract.

15. Gelmon K, Nabholtz JM, Bontebal M, et al. Randomized trial of two doses of Taxol in metastatic breast cancer after failure of standard ther-apy. Proc 8th NCI-EORTC Symposium on New Drugs in Cancer Ther-apy 1994; 8:198. Abstract.

16. Murphy WK, Fossella FV, Winn RJ, et al. Phase II study of Taxol in patients with untreated non-small-cell lung cancer. J Natl Cancer Inst 1993; 85:384–388.

17. Chang A, Kim K, Glick J, et al. Phase II study of Taxol, Merbarone, and piroxantrone in stage IV non-small-cell lung cancer: the Eastern Coop-erative Oncology Group (ECOG) results. J Natl Cancer Inst 1993; 85:388–393.

18. Forastiere A, Neuberg D, Taylor S, et al. Phase II evaluation of Taxol in advanced head and neck cancer: an Eastern Cooperative Oncology Group trial. J Natl Cancer Inst Monogr 1993; 15:181.

19. Roth BJ, Breicer R, Einhorn LH, et al. Paclitaxel in previously advanced transitional cell carcinoma of the urothelium: a Phase II trial of the Eastern Cooperative Oncology Group (ECOG). Proc Am Soc Clin Oncol 1994; 13:230. Abstract.

20. Ajani J, Ilson D, Daugherty K, et al. Activity of Taxol in patients with squamous cell carcinoma and adenocarcinoma of the esophagus. J Natl Cancer Inst 1994; 86:1086.

21. Schiff PB, Fant I, Horwitz S. Promotion of microtubule assembly in vitro by Taxol. Nature 1979; 22:665–667.

22. Parness J, Horwitz S. Taxol binds to polymerized tubulin in vitro. J Cell Biol 1981; 91:479–487.

23. Manfredi J, Parness J, Horwitz S. Taxol binds to cellular microtubules. J Cell Biol 1982; 94:688–696.

24. Wilson L. Microtubules as drug receptors: pharmacological properties of microtubule protein. Ann NY Acad Sci 1975; 253:213.

25. Carney D, Crossin K, Ball R, et al. Changes in the extent of microtubule assembly can regulate initiation of DNA synthesis. Ann NY Acad Sci 1986; 466:919.

26. Sinclair WK, Morton RA. X-ray sensitivity during the cell generation cycle of cultured Chinese hamster cells. Radiat Res 1966; 29:450–474.

27. Choy H, Rodriguez F, Koester S, et al. Investigation of Taxol as a potential radiation sensitizer. Cancer 1993; 71(11):3774–3778.

28. Geard CR, Jones JM, Schiff PB. Taxol and radiation. J Natl Cancer Inst 1993; 15:89–94.

29. Tishler R, Schiff PB, Geard C, et al. Taxol: a novel radiation sensitizer. Int J Radiat Oncol Biol Phys 1992; 22:613–617.

30. Liebmann J, Cook J, Fisher J, et al. In vitro studies of taxol as a radiation sensitizer in human tumor cells. J Natl Cancer Inst 1994; 86:441–446.

31. Minarik L, Hall E. Taxol in combination with acute and low dose rate irradiation. Radiother Oncol 1994; 32:124–128.

32. Geard C, Jones J. Radiation and Taxol on synchronized human cervical carcinoma cells. Int J Radiat Oncol Biol Phys 1994; 29:565–569.

33. Holmes F, Walters R, Theriault R, et al. Phase II trial or Taxol an active drug in the treatment of metastatic breast cancer. J Natl Cancer Inst 1991; 83:1797–1805.

34. Schiff PB, Fant J, Auster LA. Effects of Taxol on cell growth and in vitro microtubule assembly. J Supramol Struct (suppl 2) 1978; 328–335.

35. Stephens L, Ang K, Schultheiss T, et al. Apoptosis in irradiated murine tumors. Radiat Res 1991; 127:308–316.

36. Stephens L, Hunter N, Ang K, et al. Development of apoptosis irradiated murine tumors as a function of time and dose. Radiat Res 1993; 135:75–80.
37. Milas L, Hunter N, Kurdoglu B, et al. Apoptotic death of mitotically arrested cells in murine tumors treated with Taxol. Proc Am Assoc Cancer Res 1994; 35:314.
38. Meyn R, Stephens L, Hunter N, et al. Induction of apoptosis in murine tumors by cyclophosphamide. Cancer Chemother Pharmacol 1994; 33: 410–414.
39. Milas L, Hunter N, Mason K, et al. Enhancement of tumor radioresponse of a murine mammary carcinoma by paclitaxel. Cancer Res 1994; 54:3506–3510.
40. Hall EJ. Radiobiology for the Radiologist. 3rd ed. Philadelphia: J.B. Lippincott, 1988.
41. Stone HB, Milas LC, Ang KK, et al. Modification of radiation response of murine tumors. Int J Radiat Biol 1993; 64:583–591.
42. Milas L, Hunter N, Mason KA, et al. Role of rcoxygenation in induction of enhancement of tumor radioresponse by paclitaxel. Cancer Res 1995; 55:3564–3568.
43. Choy H, Akerley W, Safran H, et al. Phase I trial of outpatient weekly paclitaxel and concurrent radiation therapy for advanced non-small cell lung cancer. J Clin Oncol 1994; 14:600–609.
44. Glanz M, Choy H, Kearns M, et al. Phase I study of weekly outpatient paclitaxel and concurrent cranial irradiation in adults with astrocytomas. J Clin Oncol 1996; 12:2682–2686.
45. Choy H, Safran H. Preliminary analysis of a phase II study of weekly paclitaxel and concurrent radiation therapy for locally advanced non-small cell lung cancer. Sem Oncol 1995; 22:55–57.
46. Ansari R, Tokars R, Fisher W, et al. A Phase III study of thoracic irradiation with or without concomitant cisplatin in locoregional unresectable non small cell lung cancer (NSCLC): a Hoosier Oncology Group (H.O.G.) protocol. Proc Am Soc Clin Oncol 1991; 10:241. Abstract.
47. Kerr JFR, Winterford CM, Harmon BV. Apoptosis: its significance in cancer and cancer therapy. Cancer 1994; 73:2013–2026.
48. Lowe SW, Ruley HE, Jacks T. p53-Dependent apoptosis modulates the cytotoxicity of anticancer agents. Cell 1993; 74:957–967.
49. Lowe SW, Bodis S, McClatchey A, et al. p53 Status and the efficacy of cancer therapy in vivo. Science 1994; 266:807–810.
50. Levine AJ, Momand J, Finlay CA. The p53 tumor suppressor gene. Nature 1991; 352:453–456.

51. Naylor SL, Johnson BE, Minna JD, Sakaguchi AY. Loss of heterozygosity of chromosome 3p markers in small cell lung cancer. Nature 1987; 329:451–453.

52. Baker SJ, Fearon ER, Nigro JM, et al. Chromosome 17 deletions and p53 gene mutations in colorectal carcinomas. Science 1989; 244: 217–221.

53. Kawasaki M, Nakanisi Y, Kuwano K, Takayama K, Yatsunami J, Hara N. The utility of p53 immunostaining for the transbronchial biopsy specimens of lung cancer: p53 overexpression may predict poor prognosis and chemoresistance in advanced non-small cell lung cancer. Proc Am Soc Clin Oncol 1996; 15:94.

54. Wattel E, Prudhomme C, Hecquet B, et al. p53 Mutations are associated with resistance to chemotherapy and short survival in hematologic malignancies. Blood 1994;84:3148–3157.

55. Cohner H, Fischer K, Bentz M, et al. p53 Gene deletion predicts for poor survival and non-response to therapy with purine analogs in chronic B-cell leukemias. Blood 1995; 85:1580–1589.

56. Lenz HJ, Danenberg KD, Leichman L, et al. p53 Status and thymidylate synthase levels are predictors of chemotherapy efficacy in patients with advanced colorectal cancer. Proc Am Soc Clin Oncol 1996; 15:216.

57. Imamura J, Miyoshi I, Koeffler HP. p53 in hematologic malignancies. Blood 1994; 84:2412–2421.

58. Fung CT, Fisher D. p53 from molecular mechanism to prognosis in cancer. J Clin Oncol 1995; 13:808–811.

59. Safran H, King T, Choy H, et al. p53 Mutations do not predict response to paclitaxel radiation for nonsmall cell lung carcinoma. Cancer 1996 78:1203–1210.

60. Safran H, King T, Choy H, et al. Phase I study of paclitaxel and concurrent radiation for locally advanced gastric and pancreatic cancer. ASCO Proc 1996; 15:442.

Index

About the Editors

DAVID H. JOHNSON is Cornelius A. Craig Professor of Medical and Surgical Oncology as well as Director of the Division of Medical Oncology at Vanderbilt University School of Medicine, Nashville, Tennessee. The editor or coeditor of four books as well as the author or coauthor of nearly 200 journal papers and book chapters, Dr. Johnson is a Fellow of the American College of Physicians and a member of the American Society of Clinical Oncology, the American Association for Cancer Research, and the International Association for the Study of Lung Cancer, among others. He received the B.S. degree (1970) in zoology and the M.S. degree (1972) in physiology from the University of Kentucky, Lexington, and the M.D. degree (1976) from the Medical College of Georgia, Augusta, Georgia.

JEAN KLASTERSKY is Chairman of the Department of Medicine and Professor of Medicine, Medical Oncology, and Physical Diagnosis at the Institut Jules Bordet, Université Libre de Bruxelles, Belgium. The editor or coeditor of over 10 books, including the *Handbook of Supportive Care in Cancer* (Marcel Dekker, Inc.), and the author or coauthor of more than 340 professional papers, Dr. Klastersky is a member of the European Society for Medical Oncology, the International Association for the Study of Lung Cancer, the Infectious Diseases Society of America, the American Society of Clinical Oncology, and the American Association for Cancer Research, among others. He received the M.D. degree (1965) and the Ph.D. degree (1972) in medical sciences from the Université Libre de Bruxelles, Belgium.

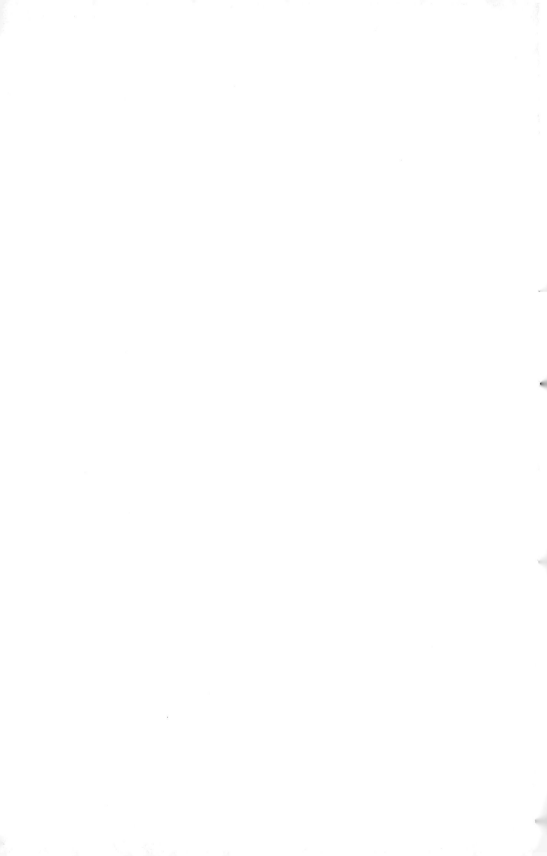